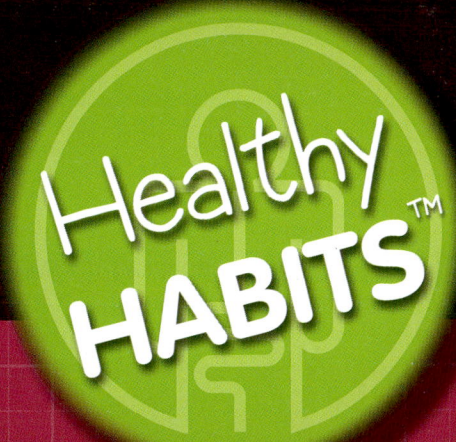

Your Immune System

Protecting Yourself Against Infection and Illness

Linda Bickerstaff

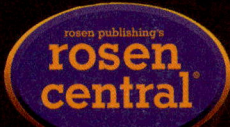

New York

Published in 2011 by The Rosen Publishing Group, Inc.
29 East 21st Street, New York, NY 10010

Copyright © 2011 by The Rosen Publishing Group, Inc.

First Edition

All rights reserved. No part of this book may be reproduced in any form without permission in writing from the publisher, except by a reviewer.

Library of Congress Cataloging-in-Publication Data

Bickerstaff, Linda.
Your immune system: protecting yourself against infection and illness / Linda Bickerstaff.—1st ed.
   p. cm.—(Healthy habits)
Includes bibliographical references and index.
ISBN 978-1-4358-9442-6 (library binding)
ISBN 978-1-4488-0612-6 (pbk)
ISBN 978-1-4488-0619-5 (6-pack)
1. Immune system. I. Title.
QR181.B48 2011
616.07'9—dc22

2009047645

Manufactured in Malaysia

CPSIA Compliance Information: Batch #S10YA: For further information, contact Rosen Publishing, New York, New York, at 1-800-237-9932.

CONTENTS

	Introduction	4
CHAPTER 1	Immune System Basics	7
CHAPTER 2	The Immune System and Infections	17
CHAPTER 3	A Healthy Diet, a Healthy Immune System	26
CHAPTER 4	Exercise and Sleep: Necessities for a Healthy Immune System	36
CHAPTER 5	Lifestyle Changes That Can Protect the Immune System	44
	Glossary	53
	For More Information	55
	For Further Reading	58
	Bibliography	60
	Index	62

Introduction

When medieval knights rode off to battle, they wore steel armor to protect themselves from arrows and swords. None of the knights knew that they were also protected by a second armor—an invisible protective shield called the immune system. This system is far more important than a suit of armor. People's immune systems protect them from the millions of bacteria, viruses, fungi, and parasites that can make them sick.

The importance of a healthy and functioning immune system is illustrated by the life and death of David Phillip Vetter. David was born in Texas in 1971 with a form of severe combined immunodeficiency disorder (SCID). SCID is an inherited malfunction of the immune system that prevents it from fighting off infections and diseases. Shortly after his birth, David was placed in a special sterile plastic "bubble" to shield him from the germs that could end his life. His story soon became front-page news in cities across the country. He became known as the "Boy in the Bubble." As David grew and developed, progressively larger bubbles were built so that he would have somewhere to live and play. Eventually, a room-sized bubble was built into his parents' home, and he was able to leave the hospital for the first time. Then he waited for medical science to find ways to treat SCID so that he could live a normal life. He waited a long time.

By the time David was twelve, his doctors had developed a new treatment that they hoped would free him from his bubble. On October 21, 1983, a small amount of bone marrow, the soft spongy material from the center of bones that makes the cells of the immune system, was taken from David's sister. It was transplanted into his body to replace his own marrow, which didn't

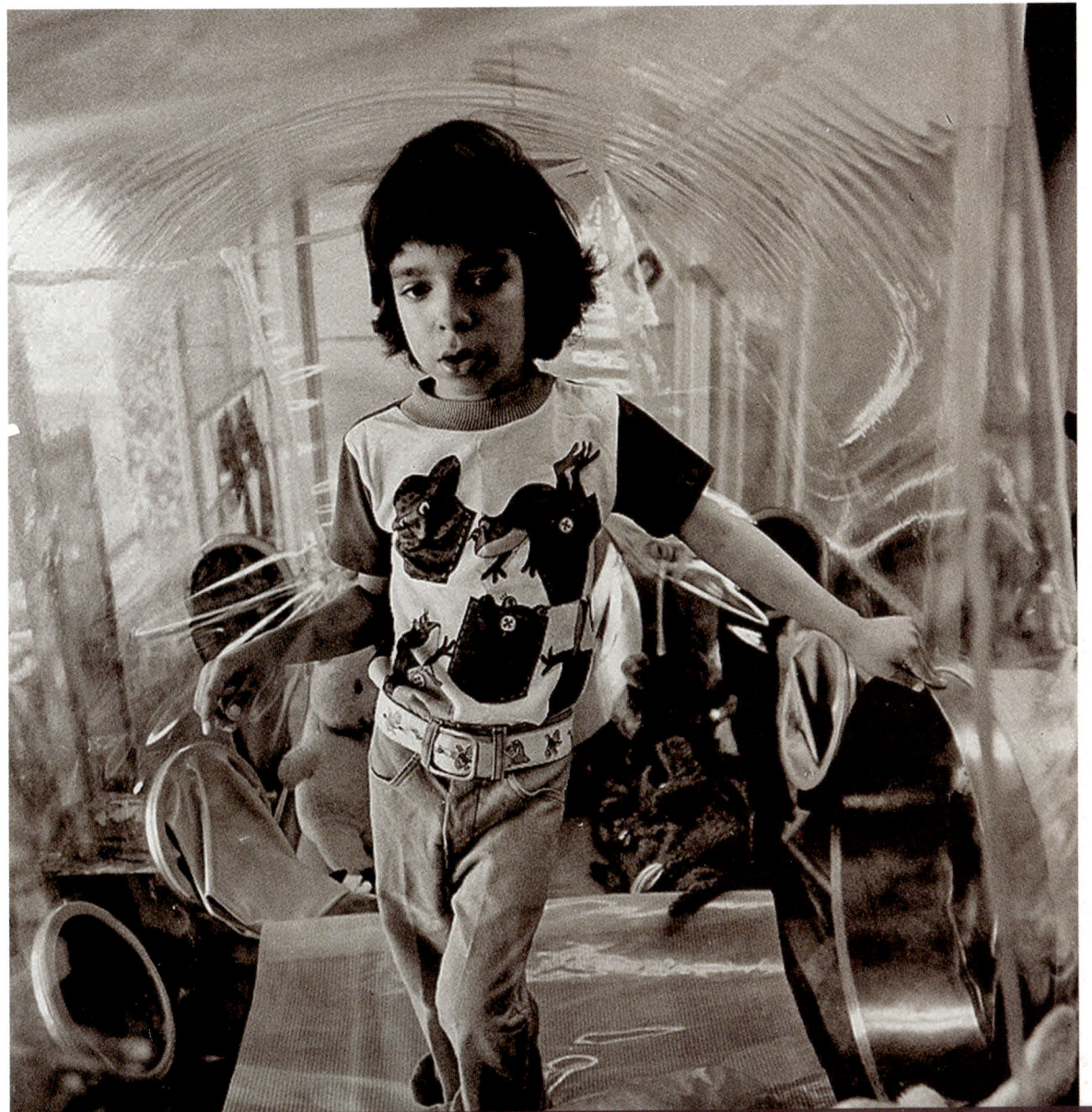
David Vetter, the "Bubble Boy," was born with severe combined immune deficiency syndrome (SCID). His immune system couldn't fight pathogens, so he had to live in a plastic bubble for protection.

make immune cells. At first, it appeared that he was cured. Soon, however, David developed a type of cancer that was caused by a virus he couldn't fight off. He died on February 22, 1984. The doctors who cared for him learned an enormous amount of information about the immune system from treating him. As his father said in an interview twenty-five years after David's death, "A lot of kids are alive today because David was here."

Few individuals are faced with problems as serious as David's, but all people face threats to their immune systems on a daily basis. The challenge that people face is keeping their immune systems healthy throughout their lifetimes. Young people are bombarded daily with advice on how to stay healthy. The amazing thing is that parents, doctors, coaches, teachers, newspaper reporters, television personalities, and even grandmothers all make the same recommendations. To stay healthy, they suggest, eat a balanced diet, get plenty of exercise and sleep, deal with stress constructively, and avoid unhealthy habits. All of these people can't be wrong. This book will look at how each of these factors helps maintain a healthy immune system to protect oneself against infection and illness.

Chapter 1

Immune System Basics

Each of the eleven organ systems of the body has a particular job to do. The immune system is the security system of the body. Its job is to protect the body from disease-causing organisms (pathogens). Because people are surrounded by billions of bacteria, fungi, parasites, and viruses that could make them sick, this is not an easy task. When threatened by these foreign invaders, a person's immune system initiates what is called an immune response to attack and kill them.

The Immune Response

Producing an immune response in the body involves many organs, specialized cells, and chemical reactions. A general description of the immune response can be broken down into the following four basic steps:

Step 1: Recognize the enemy. Each person's immune system has the ability to tell the difference between the body's own cells and foreign things that don't belong in the body. It does this by recognizing special proteins that coat every cell of a person's body. Each person has his or her own unique set of identifying proteins. Anything that is not coated with these proteins is considered

Your Immune System: Protecting Yourself Against Infection and Illness

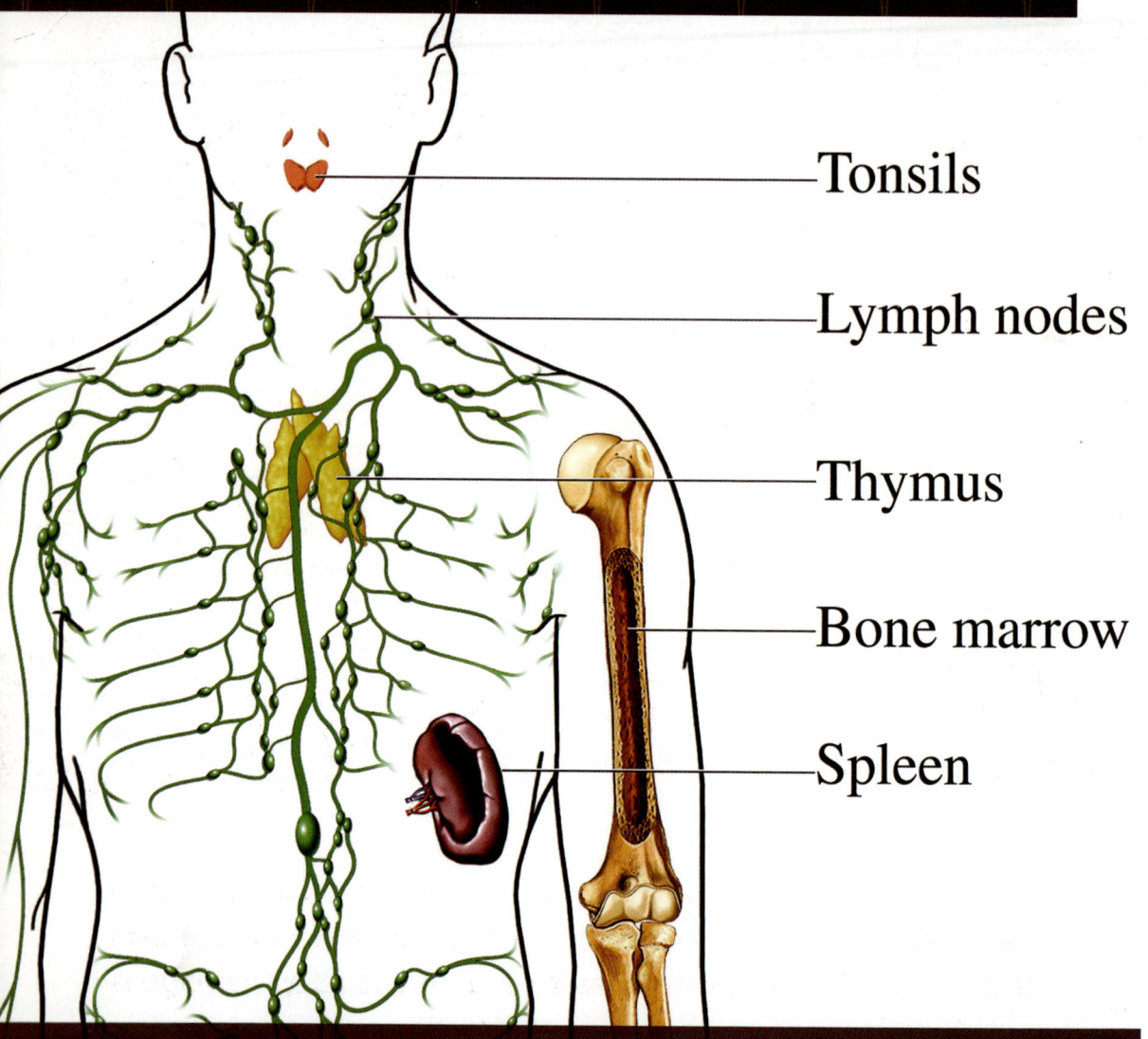

Lymph nodes, as well as the tonsils, thymus gland, spleen, and bone marrow, are all important parts of the immune system.

foreign by the immune system. Foreign substances that cause immune responses are called antigens. Bacteria, viruses, and all other pathogens are antigens. Slivers of wood, earring posts, cells from transplanted organs, and other foreign materials can also be antigens if they trigger an immune response.

Immune System Basics

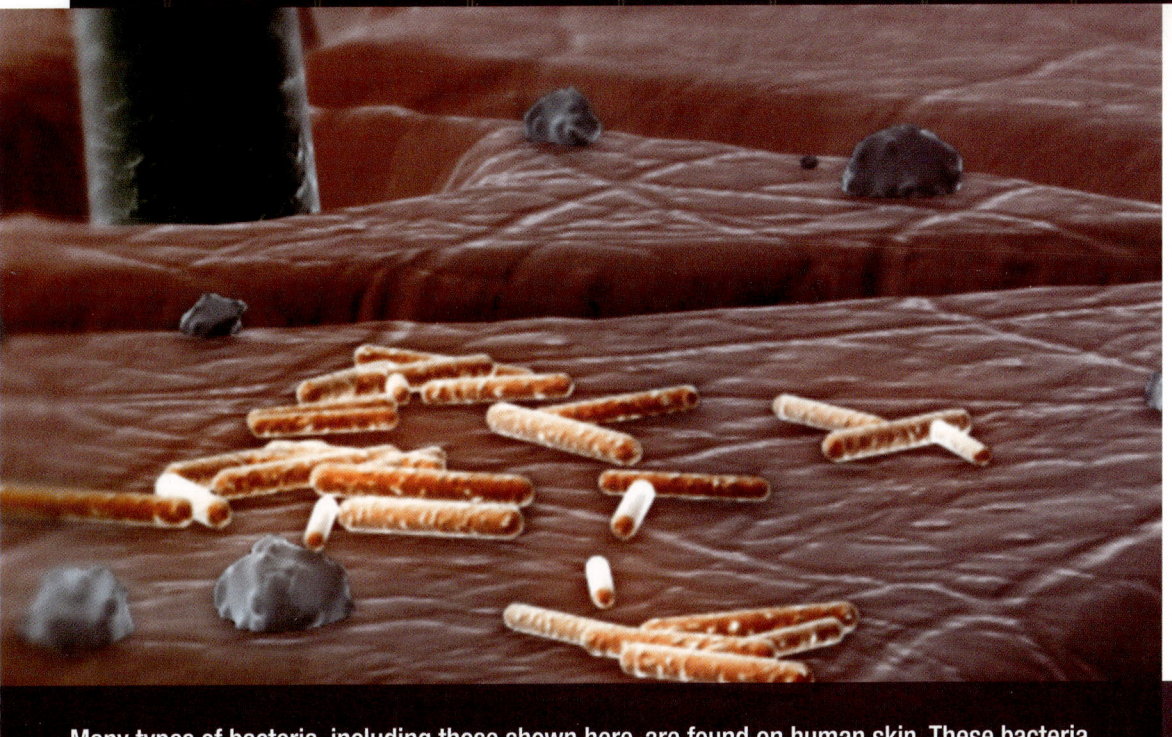

Many types of bacteria, including those shown here, are found on human skin. These bacteria usually become a problem only if the protective skin barrier breaks down or is punctured.

Step 2: Keep the enemy out. If antigens can't get into the body, they can't harm it. Like the walls around a medieval castle, the skin that surrounds the body serves as a barrier to keep pathogens out. Glands within the skin produce sweat and oil that contain chemicals that can kill bacteria. Inside the openings of the body, such as the nose and mouth, mucous membranes—not skin—provide protection. They produce a sticky substance called mucus that traps pathogens. Chemicals in mucus kill the invaders, preventing them from getting into the body. Acid in the stomach serves the same purpose. It destroys many of the pathogens found in the food and water that a person eats or drinks. The nose and other structures of the respiratory system are lined with tissues that contain large cells called macrophages. These cells can surround and eat pathogens that try to sneak into the lungs. All these organs, tissues, cells, and other structures serve as barriers to keep the enemies out.

Step 3: Respond immediately to an enemy invasion. In medieval times, invading armies that besieged a castle used battering rams to break down the castle's gates. When the gates had been shattered, the enemy invaders would rush into the castle to capture, and often kill, the people who lived there. The invaders were met by large numbers of defenders who were determined to defeat them and save the castle and its people. The immune system of the body works in a similar way. Pathogens that break through the skin or other barriers are immediately met by special defender cells. These cells are part of the immune system a person is born with, called the innate immune system. ("Innate" means existing from birth.) The information that is necessary for the immune system to recognize particular groups of pathogens is passed along from one generation to the next through genetic material. Using this inborn information, a person's innate immune system can respond immediately to these pathogens.

Consider what happens if a person gets a splinter in his or her finger. When the splinter pierces the skin, the bacteria that are located on the skin are pushed deep into the tissue of the finger. The passage of the splinter through the tissues damages many tissue cells. The damaged cells release cytokines, which are chemicals that switch on the innate immune system. Once it is switched on, the innate immune system sends defender cells to battle the bacteria that it already knows can be dangerous. The defender cells are types of white blood cells that are made in the bone marrow. When they are mature, they are carried in the blood to areas in the body where they are needed. When they are released into tissues around the

Immune System Basics

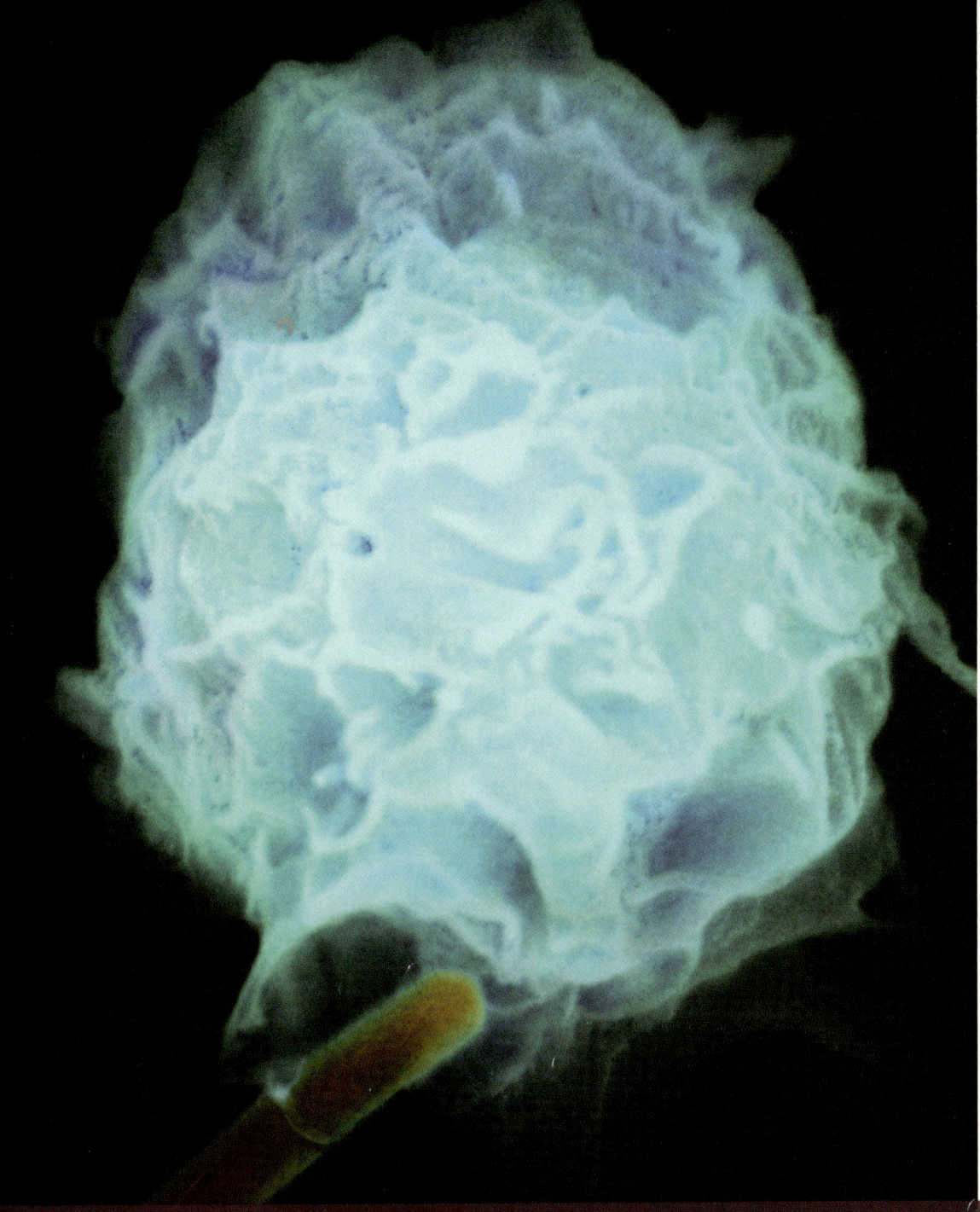

One of the defender cells of the innate immune system is the macrophage. This picture shows a macrophage (blue cell) "eating" a bacterium (orange rod) that has invaded the body.

splinter, some of the cells "eat" all the pathogens that they can find. Other defender cells kill bacteria with chemicals. In the process, some of the chemicals from these cells leak out into the tissues. These chemicals cause the person's finger to get hot, red, swollen, and sore. This reaction is called inflammation. It is evidence that the innate immune system is working.

Step 4: Build a better defense system. There are some pathogens that the innate immune system is not preprogrammed to attack. The innate immune system can slow these invaders down, but it can't kill them. Fortunately, there is a backup system, called the acquired immune system. People are not born with acquired immunity. They develop it throughout their lives as they are exposed to antigens. This system is switched on at the same time that the innate system is triggered. It takes at least seven days, however, before it is ready to help defend the body. White blood cells called lymphocytes are the defenders in this system. They are also made in the bone marrow. Some of them stay there until they are mature. These are called B lymphocytes, or B cells. Other lymphocytes migrate out of the marrow while they are immature and travel to the thymus gland. There, they mature into either killer T cells or helper T cells.

The job of B cells is to produce proteins called antibodies. B cells are similar to a tailor who uses a pattern to make a suit of clothes. B cells use antigens as the patterns to make antibodies. (Each B cell is programmed to make a particular antibody.) When the antibodies have been made, they fit perfectly over the antigens and attach to them. Once the B cells coat the antigens with their specific antibodies, helper T cells can recognize that the antigens are dangerous to the body. They send killer T cells to destroy these antigens. B cells also "remember" the antigens against which

To Pierce or Not to Pierce

Although body piercing has existed for thousand of years, it is now a fashion statement in the United States. Today, body parts from head to toe display jewelry. With rare exceptions, an innate immune response occurs when a foreign object, such as a belly or nose ring, breaks through the skin or mucous membranes. The result is inflammation. The sites around the inserted jewelry become hot, red, swollen, and sore. Inflammation may last from weeks to months before the puncture sites heal. Areas of the body such as the nose, lips, and tongue harbor huge numbers of bacteria. When these areas are pierced, a person not only develops inflammation, but is also at high risk for getting an infection. There may be more bacteria pushed past the barriers of the skin and mucous membranes than the immune system can fight off.

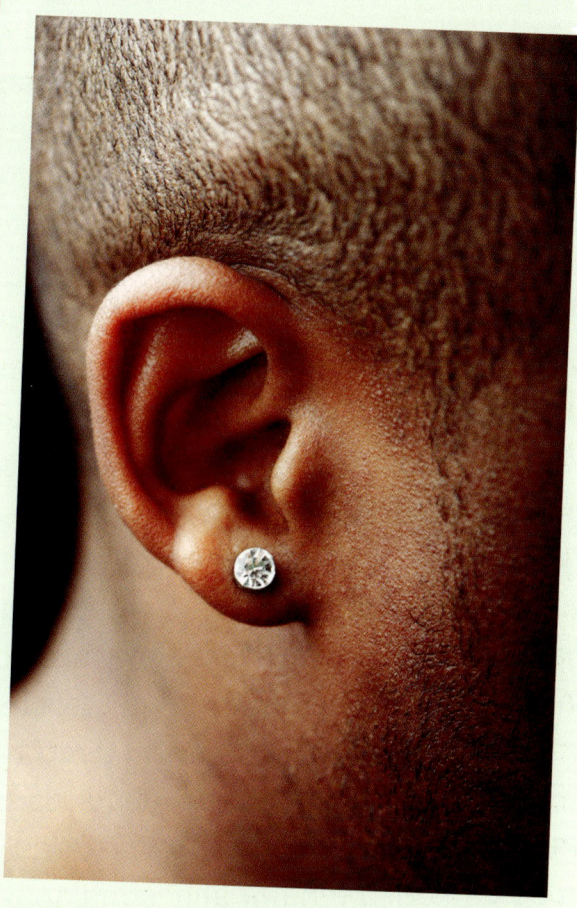

An innate immune response occurs when foreign bodies, such as earring posts, pierce the skin. Here, slight swelling of the boy's earlobe reflects this immune response.

they have made antibodies. The next time the body is exposed to those antigens, antibodies are already present in the bloodstream, and the "memory" B cells can quickly make even more of these antibodies.

Immune System Failures

Even the immune system can break down. When it does, people develop conditions or illnesses because it fails to function properly. These conditions are called disorders. Immune system disorders are classified into the following four groups.

Immunodeficiency Disorders

If the immune system fails to do its job of protecting a person against pathogens, that person may have an immunodeficiency disorder. Some children, like the "Boy in the Bubble," inherit abnormal genes that keep their immune systems from working properly from birth. These children have primary immunodeficiency disorders. According to medical researchers at the Mayo Clinic, a well-known medical organization based in Rochester, Minnesota, there are more than one hundred different primary immunodeficiency disorders. These disorders affect at least fifty thousand people in the United States.

People can also develop secondary or acquired immunodeficiency disorders later in life. For instance, a person's immune system can be damaged if he or she is malnourished or is badly burned in a fire. Some of the drugs that are used to treat patients who have cancer or who have received organ transplants can also harm the immune system. Even some viral infections, such as those caused by the human immunodeficiency virus (HIV), can cause immunodeficiency disorders.

Autoimmune Disorders

Autoimmune disorders occur if the immune system mistakes a person's own body cells for foreign cells and makes antibodies against them. These healthy cells are then destroyed, just like they would have been if they had been foreign invaders. One autoimmune disorder that occurs in children and teens is juvenile rheumatoid arthritis. Cells from the joints of young people who have this disorder are mistaken for foreign cells. As the healthy cells are attacked and killed by the immune system, the young person's joints can become deformed.

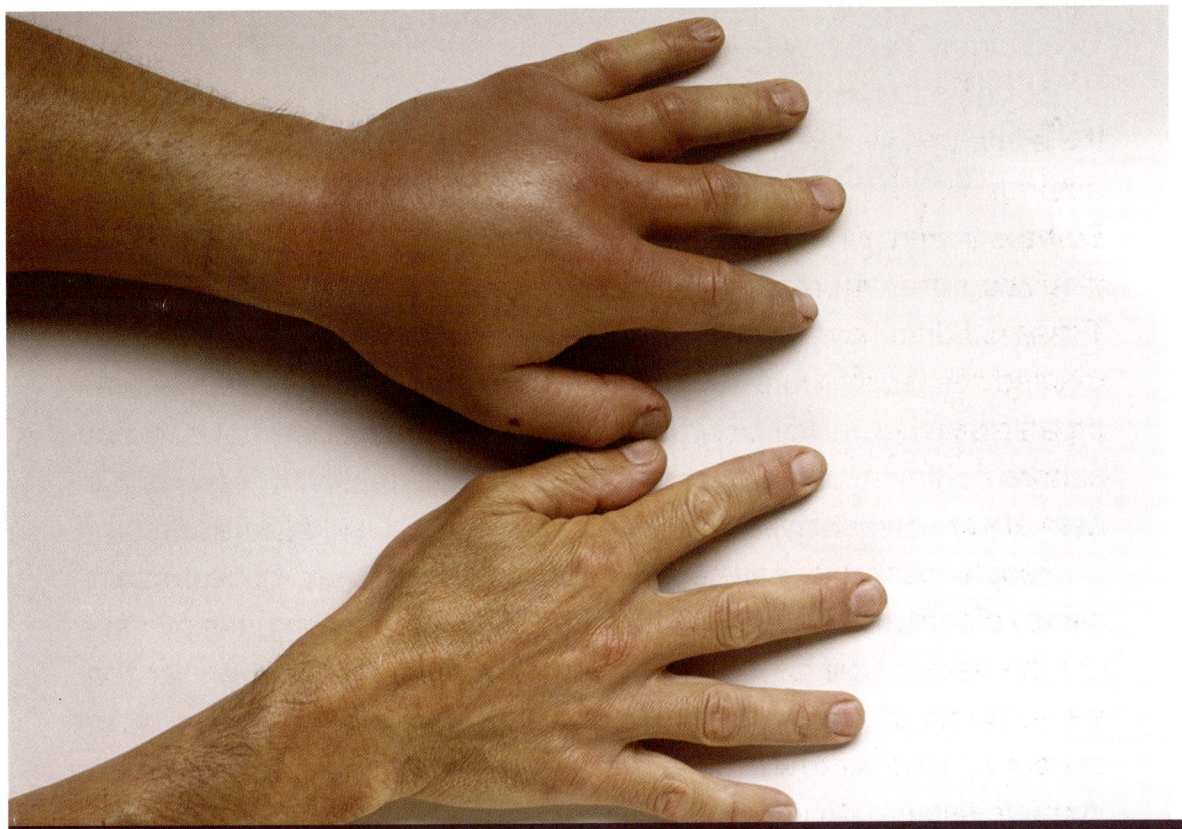

Some people develop allergies to bee-sting venom. The swelling seen in this man's left hand is the result of such an allergy. Bee stings can be fatal to some allergic individuals.

Allergies

Allergies occur if the immune system overreacts to contact with antigens in the environment. The immune system mistakes harmless environmental substances, such as house mold or dust mites, for harmful pathogens and builds antibodies against them. Substances that cause allergic responses are called allergens.

Hay fever and other seasonal allergies result when the immune system makes antibodies against pollens. These allergies are relatively common, and their symptoms are usually mild. Some people develop allergies that can be life threatening, though. For instance, people may develop allergies to peanuts, shellfish, or bee stings that, if not treated promptly, can be deadly.

Cancers of the Immune System

Cancer occurs when cells begin to grow in an unregulated way. They don't mature into cells that function normally. They can invade healthy tissues. Cancers of the white blood cells are called leukemias. They are the most common types of cancer in children. Related cancers can also occur in lymphoid tissue, such as the spleen and lymph nodes, and are called lymphomas. They are relatively common in teens and young adults. Fortunately, childhood leukemia and some types of lymphomas can be treated successfully. Many children and teens with these cancers can be cured.

Although some immune system disorders cannot be prevented, most can now be treated. Some immune system failures can be avoided by a person's actions. Later chapters in this book will look at what a person can do to maintain a healthy immune system and maximize its function.

Chapter 2

The Immune System and Infections

All people live in a sea of bacteria. There are bacteria in water, food, and the air that each person breathes. Bacteria reside on every square inch of a person's skin. They are also found throughout people's respiratory and digestive systems. In addition, humans are surrounded by millions of virus particles, fungi, and parasites. People manage to live in harmony with most of these microorganisms and even benefit from many of them. A healthy immune system makes all this possible. If the immune system fails, microorganisms that are normally harmless can become pathogens and cause serious health problems.

What Is an Infection?

An infection occurs when a pathogen invades a person's body and begins to multiply in body tissues. If the infection is bad enough, the person's cells are damaged or destroyed. That person then has a disease. The signs and symptoms of the infection or disease vary depending on what organism is causing the infection. Signs and symptoms might be a drippy nose, a sore throat, a cough, or a red and swollen finger or other body part. The symptoms, though, are not caused by the pathogens themselves. They result when the immune

Your Immune System: Protecting Yourself Against Infection and Illness

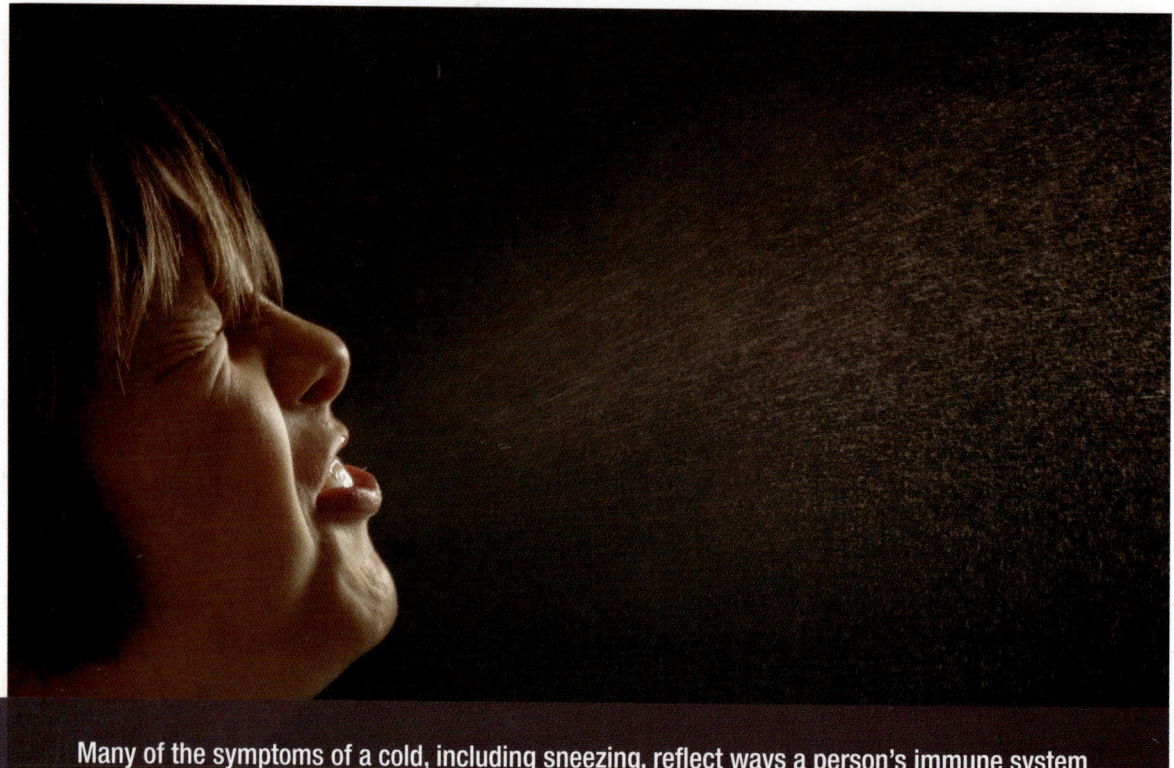

Many of the symptoms of a cold, including sneezing, reflect ways a person's immune system attempts to rid the body of viruses that cause infections.

system begins to fight the infection. For example, a person who gets a cold develops a drippy nose and has a lot of sneezing and coughing. These symptoms reflect ways that the immune system is trying to rid the body of the viruses that are causing the infection. The drippy nose occurs because the immune system stimulates cells in the nose to increase their production of mucus. Mucus traps viruses before they can cause trouble. Sneezing also helps rid the nose of viruses. Coughing keeps mucus, which has trapped viruses, from getting into the lungs. The elevated temperature that a person sometimes develops with influenza (flu) is also part of an immune response. Most human pathogens do not tolerate temperatures much higher than normal body temperature (98.6 degrees Fahrenheit, or 37 degrees Celsius). If a person's temperature gets up to 101 or 102°F (38 or 39°C), many pathogens will die. When a person's temperature drops to normal, he or she is probably on the road to recovery from the infection.

Viral Infections Versus Bacterial Infections

Only about 1 percent of bacteria cause infections in humans. Almost all viruses do, however. The reason for this is that bacteria are one-celled organisms that can grow and reproduce on their own. They can live on a person's skin or in the mucous membranes without causing injury to those structures. Viruses, on the other hand, are not cells. They are tiny bundles of genetic material, either deoxyribonucleic acid (DNA) or ribonucleic acid (RNA). Viruses are incapable of living on their own. They must invade body cells to get the food and energy that they need to grow and reproduce. Viruses eventually kill the cells that they invade.

Viral infections tend to spread more easily from person to person than do bacterial infections. An upper respiratory tract infection (a cold), for instance, is the most common viral infection among all people in the United States. There are more than two hundred types of viruses that can cause colds. They cause more than one billion infections in the United States each year. Pediatricians estimate that children get between three and eight colds every year. Cold viruses are spread in several ways. They are propelled into the air when a person sneezes or coughs. They can also be picked up if a person touches something that is contaminated and then touches his or her face, nose, mouth, or eyes.

Your Immune System: Protecting Yourself Against Infection and Illness

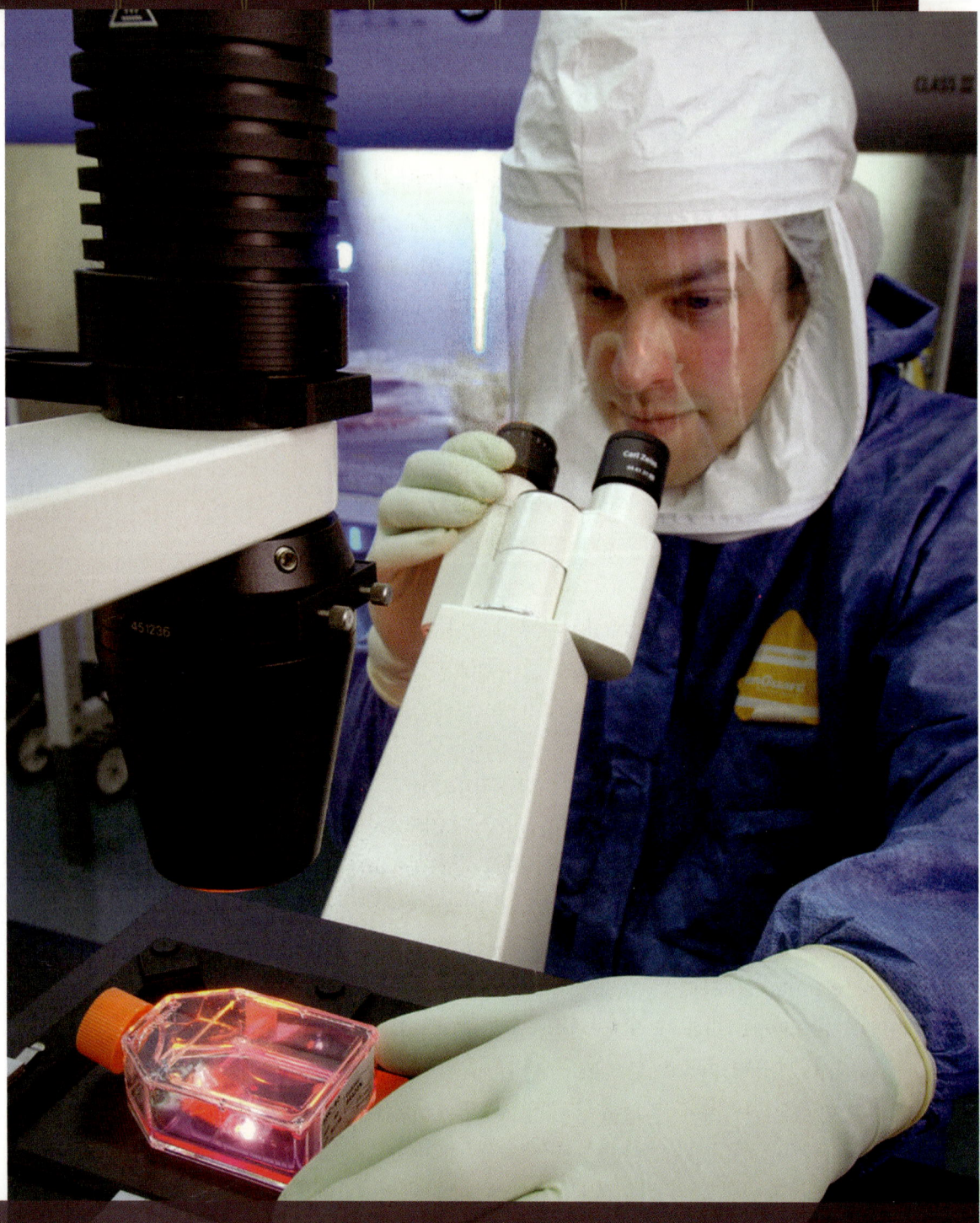

A medical researcher is shown here making vaccines against influenza viruses. Being vaccinated usually protects a person against the viruses contained in the vaccine.

The immune system is the only defense a person has against viral infections. Although a few antiviral drugs have been developed, viruses mutate, or change, so rapidly that these drugs are not effective for very long. Infections caused by viruses that are new to a person's body may take a long time to resolve because antibodies must be made against the viruses before T cells can kill them. Bacterial infections, on the other hand, can be treated with antibiotics. Getting this kind of treatment means that the immune system does not have to work so hard. With a proper course of antibiotics, a bacterial infection can usually be cleared up relatively quickly.

Prevention Is Worth a Pound of Cure

Doctors say the best way to stay disease-free is to prevent infections from occurring in the first place. They recommend the following steps for avoiding infections:

- Frequent hand washing. Washing hands before preparing or eating food, after coughing or sneezing, or after using the toilet is the single most important step that a person can take to prevent an infection. In the absence of water, use alcohol-based hand-sanitizing gels to clean hands.
- Keep vaccinations current. A vaccine is a fluid that contains a small amount of a specific type of viral or bacterial material. If some of the fluid is injected under a person's skin, his or her immune system builds antibodies against the pathogens that are contained in the vaccine. When the person is exposed to the pathogens again, antibodies that are lying in wait will kill the pathogens before they can cause illness. Almost all children in the United States are immunized against several organisms

Your Immune System: Protecting Yourself Against Infection and Illness

that can cause serious infections. Infections such as measles, mumps, chickenpox, whooping cough, and poliomyelitis have almost been eliminated among children in the United States because they have been vaccinated against them.

- Take medications to prevent some infections before they even occur. Some infectious diseases, such as malaria, are very difficult to cure. If a person is going to travel to a region of the world where malaria occurs, it is recommended that the person take medication for protection against the parasite that causes it in case he or she is exposed.

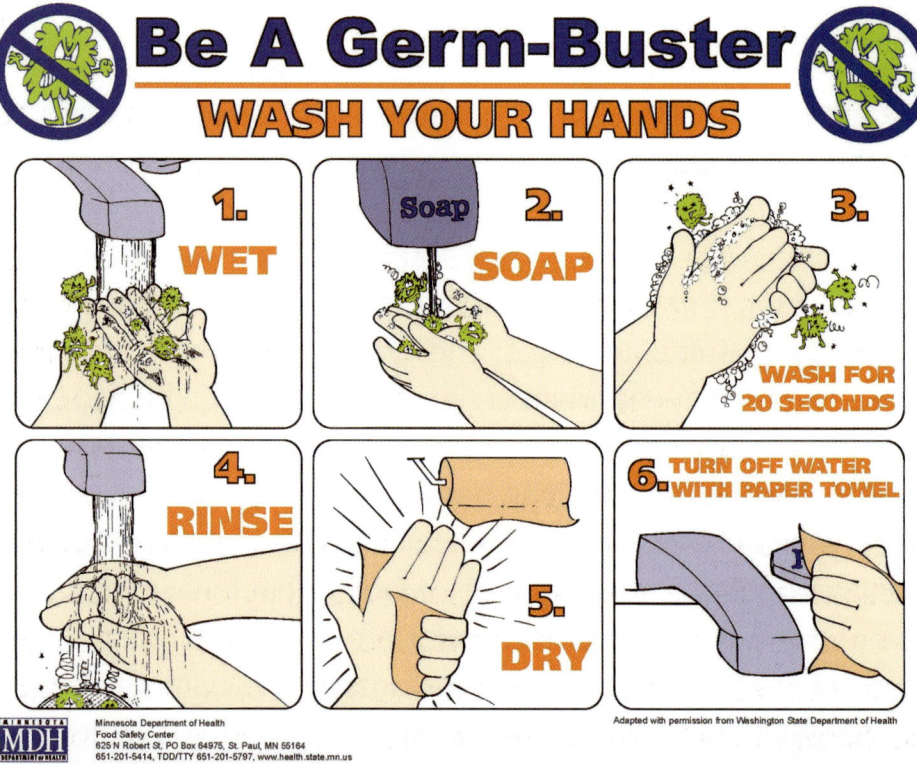

It is better to prevent infections than to try to cure them. Frequent, thorough hand washing is the most important way to help prevent infections.

Antibiotic-Resistant Bacteria

Penicillin was the first antibiotic to be discovered. It was found to be particularly effective in killing two types of bacteria commonly found in and on the human body. The bacteria *Streptococcus* and *Staphylococcus* cause a significant number of the infections that humans get. Shortly after they started to use penicillin to treat infections, scientists noted that some staphylococci were not killed by the drug. They called these penicillin-resistant staphylococci. Today, almost every bacterial pathogen has developed resistance to one or more of the antibiotics that were previously used to kill it. Alarmingly, a few bacteria are resistant to all antibiotics. Combinations of very strong antibiotics are the only ways to kill these organisms.

The following are some of the factors that scientists believe contribute to the development of antibiotic-resistant bacteria:

- Inappropriate use of antibiotics. Antibiotics will not kill viruses, but they are frequently given to people who have viral infections. Before doctors realized how quickly bacteria can mutate and what a problem antibiotic-resistant bacteria can be, they were less cautious about prescribing antibiotics than they are now.
- Failure to take all of the antibiotic pills that were prescribed. When people who have been given antibiotics for an infection start to feel better, they often decide that they do not need to continue taking the antibiotics that doctors have prescribed for them. As a result, an infection may be inadequately treated and the bacteria that cause the infection can develop antibiotic resistance. The infection may return several days after the antibiotics are stopped. More antibiotics, or a different antibiotic, must then be taken.

Clean Hands Are Cool Hands

Mitchel Musso, who plays Hannah Montana's cool sidekick Oliver Oken in the Disney TV series *Hannah Montana*, is the spokesperson for a campaign sponsored by the Hospital Corporation of America. The goal of the campaign is to teach young people and their parents how important good hand washing is in preventing infections. The actor participated in public service announcements on television and made personal appearances at several schools across the country to spread the word that "Clean Hands Are Cool Hands." The campaign was originally launched to fight the spread of methicillin-resistant *Staphylococcus aureus* (MRSA), a bacterial infection that is causing many infections among schoolchildren. It has since been extended to emphasis the importance of good hand washing in preventing the spread of H1N1 influenza, or swine flu. Check out the Clean Hands Are Cool Hands Web site, http://www.cleanhandsarecoolhands.com, to see what Musso has to say about the importance of hand washing.

- Failure to take the medication as directed. The number of times an antibiotic pill must be taken each day varies with the antibiotic. If a person fails to take the antibiotic as directed, the drug may not be effective in curing that person's infection.
- The use of antibiotics in animal feed to promote the growth of animals. More than 70 percent of antibiotics used in the United States are mixed into animal feed. Meat producers know that animals that receive antibiotics in their food are larger and healthier than those that don't. Meat producers use the same antibiotics that doctors prescribe for people who have bacterial infections. As a result, the wide use of antibiotics in animal

The Immune System and Infections

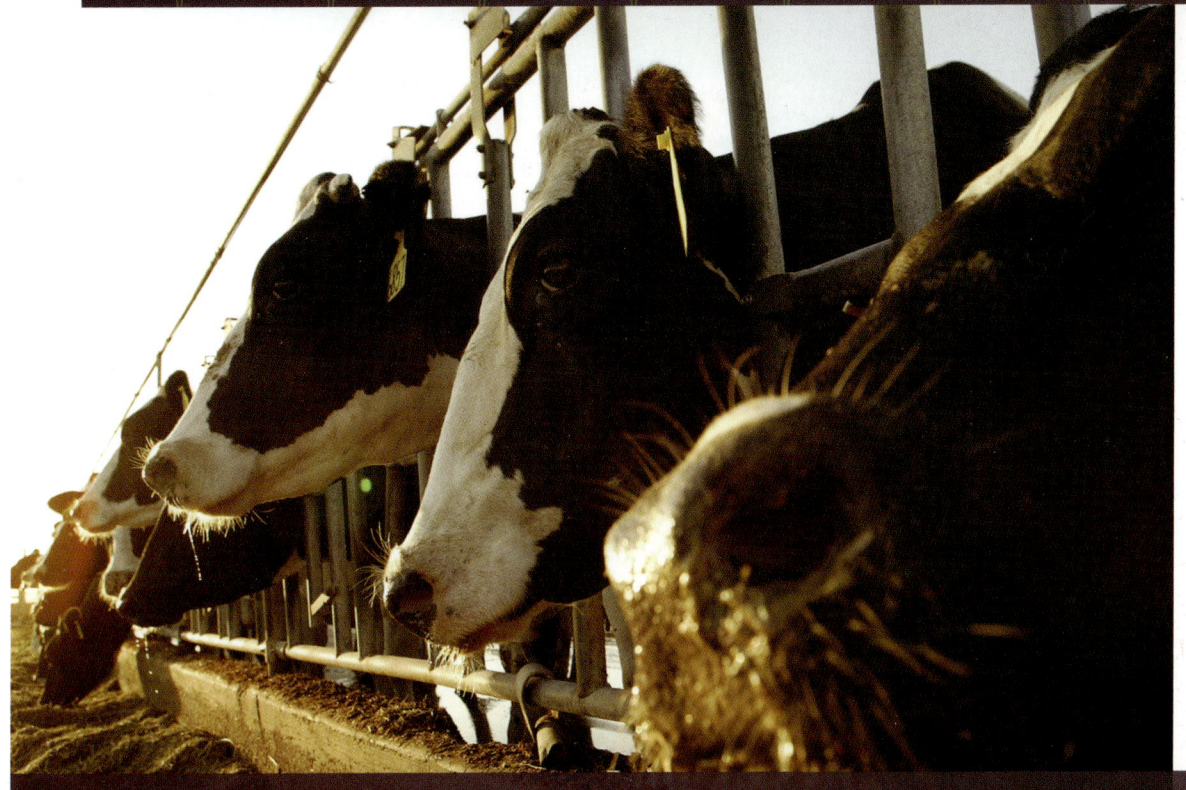

Seventy percent of the antibiotics used in the United States are found in animal food. This widespread use of antibiotics has increased the rate of development of antibiotic-resistant strains of bacteria.

feed has increased the rate of the development of antibiotic-resistant strains of bacteria.

Bacteria that are strong enough to resist the effects of antibiotics survive to pass on their genetic traits to future generations of bacteria. Although scientists have not found a magic cure that will wipe out these "superbugs," they are making great progress in investigating new methods of treatment.

Chapter 3

A Healthy Diet, a Healthy Immune System

German philosopher Ludwig Feuerbach (1804–1872) once said, "Man is what he eats." Exactly what Feuerbach meant is unknown. He may have meant that what people eat affects how healthy they are. To stay healthy, people need to have an immune system that works properly. Therefore, they need to eat foods that will give the immune system all the nutrients it needs in order to do its job. It doesn't take special foods, vitamin pills, or expensive supplements to get these nutrients. What it takes is the balanced diet that many people in the United States eat every day.

Elements of a Balanced Diet

A balanced diet is one that supplies a proper amount of all the nutrients that a person needs to remain healthy. Some nutrients are especially important for the health of the immune system. Proteins provide part of the energy that the immune system needs to do its job. Proteins are made of building blocks called amino acids. When proteins are digested, the amino acids are absorbed into the body. They are used to help repair body parts and help with growth. Amino acids are essential for the production of the millions of white blood cells that the immune system needs to do its work.

A Healthy Diet, a Healthy Immune System

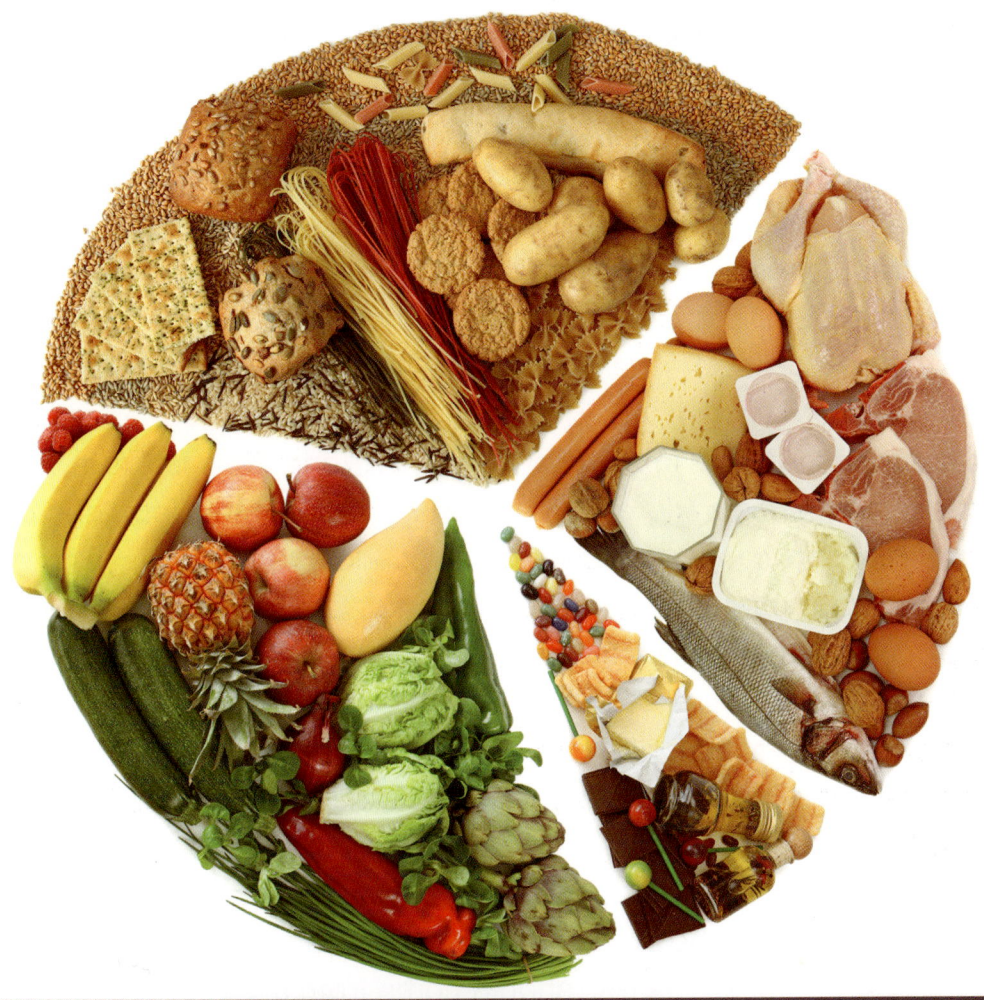

The elements of a balanced diet are depicted in this picture. All of the nutrients a person needs to maintain a healthy immune system are contained in a balanced diet.

Protein-energy malnutrition is the most common cause of immune system failure worldwide.

Nutritionists recommend that a person eat .02 to .03 of an ounce (0.8 to 1.0 gram) of protein for every 2.2 pounds (1 kilogram) of body weight. For example, if a person weighs 100 pounds (45.4 kg), he or she should eat between 1.3 and 1.6 ounces (36 and 45 grams) of protein each day. Most of the protein eaten should come from sources that contain little fat, such as seafood, skinless chicken or turkey, eggs, beans, lentils, and soy products.

Proper amounts of fat are also needed for good functioning of the immune system. Fat is a source of energy for the immune system. Some types of fat are harmful to the heart and blood vessels, so their use should be limited. These harmful fats are saturated fats (for example, those found in butter and red meat) and trans fats (like those in vegetable shortening and margarine). Unsaturated fats, such as those found in canola oil, olive oil, avocados, nuts, and seeds, are good energy sources and are less harmful. Omega-3 fatty acids are also good sources of energy. They are found in fish like salmon, tuna, and sardines. Diets that contain adequate amounts of unsaturated fats boost immune function by making T cells work more efficiently. On the other hand, diets that are high in saturated fats impair immune system response by decreasing the function of T cells. Nutritionists recommend that only 30 percent of the calories a person consumes each day be from fat. Of the 30 percent, only 5 to 10 percent should come from saturated fats. The rest should come from unsaturated fats.

Carbohydrates serve as a very important energy source for the immune system. During digestion, carbohydrates are broken down into sugars that can be absorbed and used to supply energy. The bodies of people who don't eat enough carbohydrates begin to break down proteins in order to get energy. This effect robs the immune system of the amino acids that are needed to make immune cells. It is recommended that simple sugars, such as those found in soft drinks, candy, and many other foods that young people enjoy, be eaten only in small quantities. Complex carbohydrates provide the same energy in a more healthful way. They are found in breads, cereals, potatoes, and many other types of food.

The immune system simply doesn't work without several vitamins, minerals, and trace elements. These substances are called micronutrients because they are only needed in small quantities. The ones that are most important to the immune system are vitamin A, several of the B vitamins, and vitamins C and E. Other necessary micronutrients are folic acid, iron, zinc, and selenium. Deficiencies of any of the vitamins can affect white blood cell production and function.

Many micronutrients can actually be harmful to the immune system if they are taken in large quantities. Although vitamins, minerals, and trace elements can be obtained in pill form from pharmacies and health-food stores, they are expensive and often poorly absorbed

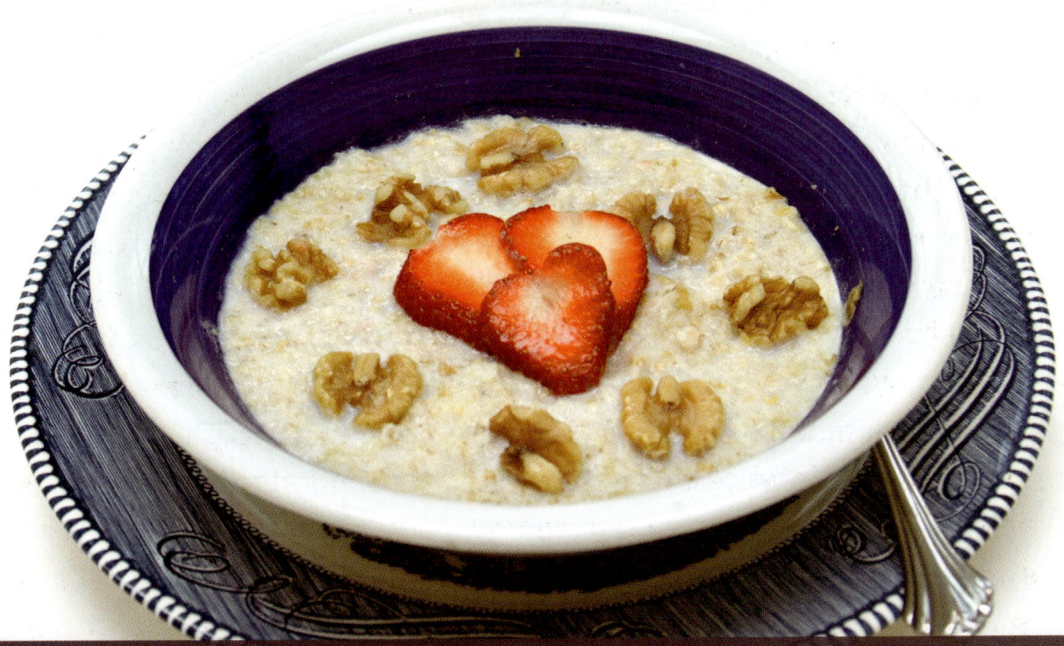

Complex carbohydrates, such as those found in this bowl of oatmeal, are important sources of energy for the immune system.

into a person's body. If a doctor recommends that a person take a particular vitamin each day, he or she should follow that recommendation. Otherwise, eat five to nine servings of fruits and vegetables each day. This amount provides more than enough vitamins, minerals, and trace elements to meet a person's daily needs.

Popeye Was No Dummy!

Popeye the Sailor Man, a cartoon character created in 1929 by Elzie Crisler Segar, was really smart. He knew that spinach gave him the superhuman strength that he needed to do all of his heroic deeds. It also helped him rescue his sweetheart, Olive Oyl, from the clutches of the villain, Bluto. What Popeye may not have known was how important spinach was to his immune system. Spinach and other green, leafy vegetables such as mustard greens and Swiss chard offer more micronutrients than any other foods. Spinach itself contains more than eighty nutrients, including most of those needed for a healthy immune system. Popeye usually ate canned spinach. He squeezed a spinach can until it popped open and then sucked the spinach through his corncob pipe and right into his mouth. Had Popeye known that fresh spinach, or lightly steamed spinach, contained more nutrients than canned spinach, he would have probably pulled spinach right out of the ground and eaten it raw!

The Effects of Obesity on the Immune System

Obesity is one of the greatest health problems in the United States for both children and adults. Being overweight injures all body

A Healthy Diet, a Healthy Immune System

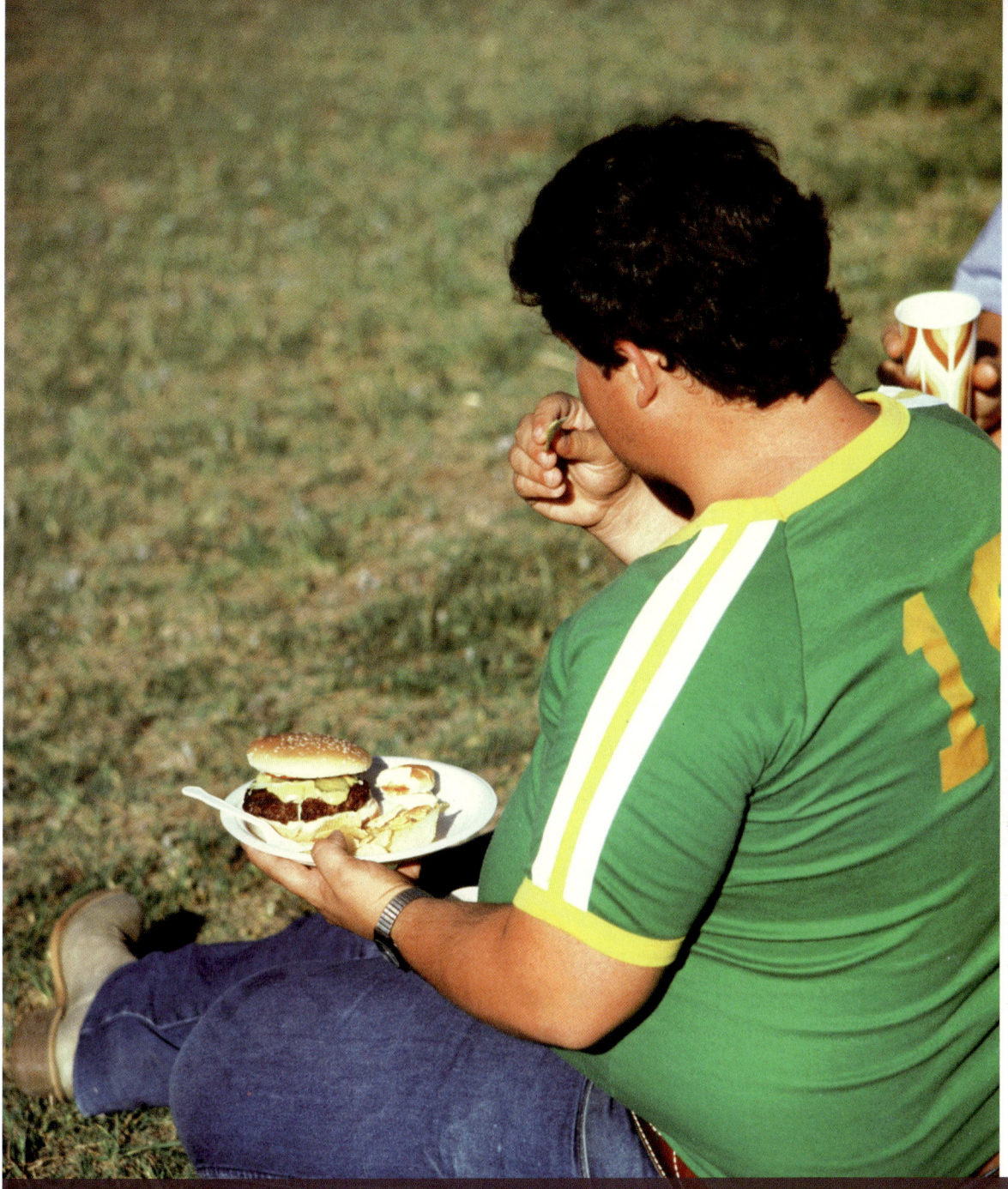

Obesity is one of the greatest health problems among teens in the United States. Those who are overweight get more infections than do those of normal weight and do not heal as well.

systems, including the immune system. Scientific studies using obese mice show that they are not able to fight off infections as easily as mice of normal weight. It has also been observed that people who are overweight have a much harder time healing wounds. They get more infections than people of average weight who are exposed to the same pathogens. Researchers think that poor cytokine function may be the key to these problems. Cytokines are the chemical substances released from injured cells that start the immune response. Some cytokines also stimulate B cells to make antibodies. If cytokines don't work correctly, the immune system is slow to react to pathogens, and foreign invaders can get a good foothold in the body before the immune system knows they are there.

Food Allergies, an Immune System Mistake

Although many people think that they have food allergies, few really do. About 6 percent of American children have food allergies. Most of these allergies disappear as children get older. With food allergies, the immune system mistakes a harmless substance, such as a peanut, for a foreign invader. It makes antibodies against this allergen. When a person eats more peanuts, an immune response occurs—a chemical called histamine is released into the person's body. Histamine usually causes mild symptoms, such as an itchy nose and sneezing or watery eyes. In some people, symptoms can be much more severe and even life threatening. For example, a person might have serious trouble breathing and will need emergency medication to help him or her breathe more easily.

The best, and sometimes only, way to treat food allergies is to avoid eating the foods that cause them. Eggs, milk, peanuts, and tree

A Healthy Diet, a Healthy Immune System

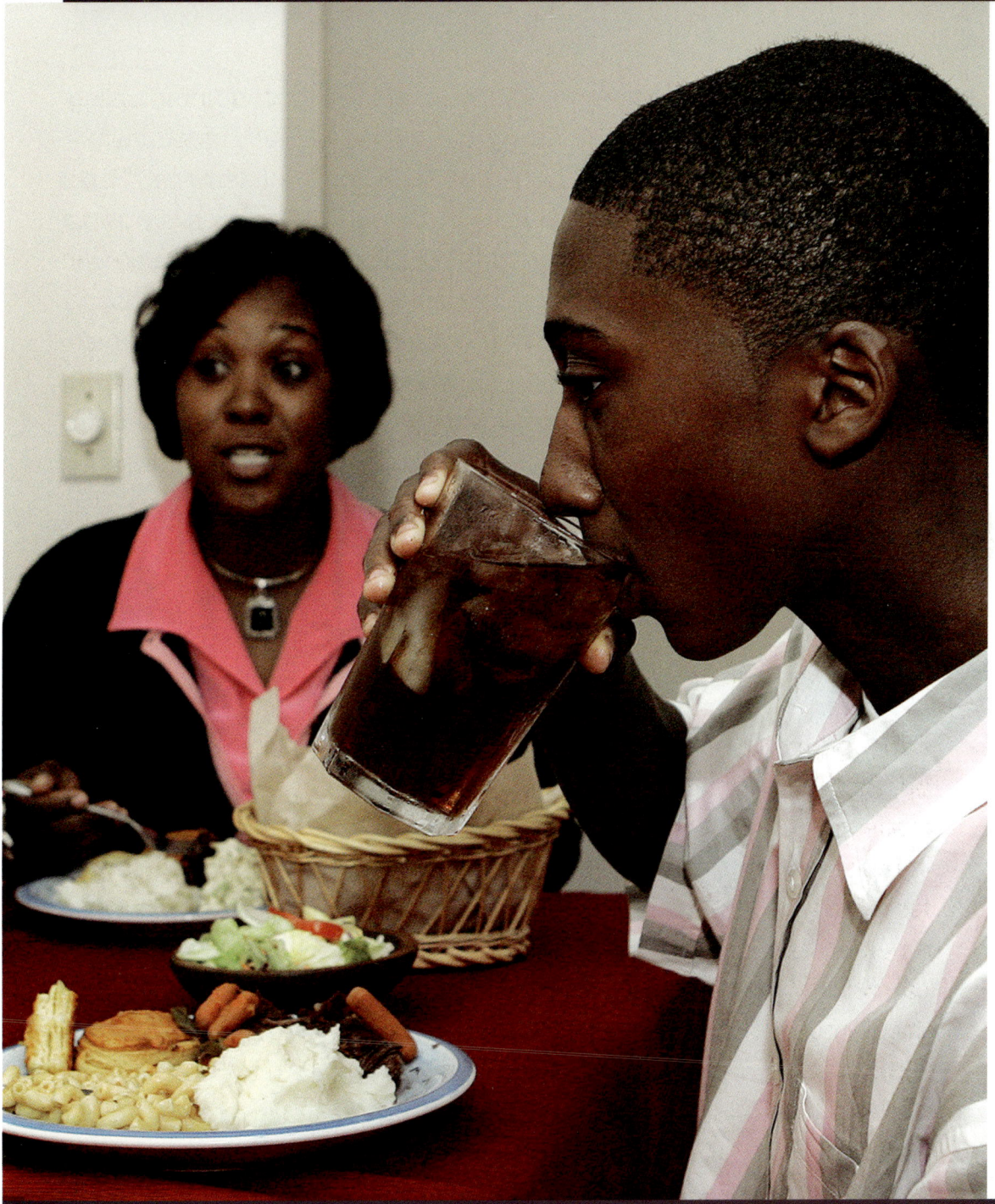

The teenager shown here with his mother cannot drink milk or eat ice cream. He is lactose intolerant and therefore cannot digest products containing the milk sugar, lactose.

nuts (walnuts and cashews, for example) are the most common allergens that affect children.

Food allergies are often confused with food intolerance. Food intolerance usually occurs because a person lacks an enzyme to properly digest food. Allergic reactions occur almost immediately, whereas the symptoms of food intolerance occur several minutes to hours after eating. An example of food intolerance is lactose intolerance. Lactose is the sugar found in milk. Many people do not have the enzyme lactase in their intestines, which is necessary to digest lactose. As a result, they develop abdominal pain and diarrhea after drinking milk or eating cheese or ice cream.

MYTHS and FACTS

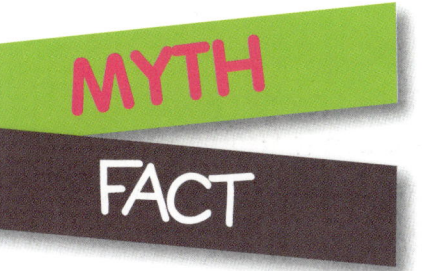

As long as antibiotics are available, people don't have to worry about infections.

Only bacterial infections can be treated with antibiotics. Many infections are caused by viruses, fungi, and parasites. These do not respond to antibiotics. In general, a healthy immune system is much more important than antibiotics in controlling most infections.

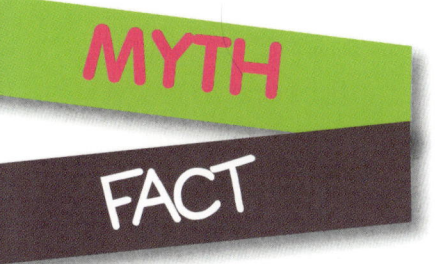

The most important way to prevent infections is to take antibiotics.

Good hand washing is the best way to keep from getting an infection.

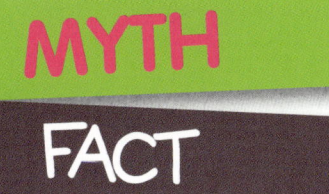

Taking pills that contain vitamins, minerals, and other micronutrients is necessary to maintain a healthy immune system.

All the micronutrients a person needs can be obtained from fruits and vegetables. It is better to get micronutrients from food than from pills because they are absorbed from food more easily and completely. Some supplement pills may contain so much of these micronutrients that they can actually harm the immune system.

Chapter 4

Exercise and Sleep: Necessities for a Healthy Immune System

Getting plenty of exercise and sleep are as important to the maintenance of a healthy immune system as eating a balanced diet. Doctors, fitness trainers, and even coaches have long observed that people who get regular exercise get fewer infections. This is especially true of colds and the flu, which involve the upper part of the respiratory system. Why those who exercise regularly get fewer infections has been a mystery until recently. Researchers in the area of exercise immunology are finding the answers to this mystery. There is also much research being done on how sleep affects the immune system.

Exercise and the Immune System

Several scientific studies have shown that people who exercise regularly have fewer infections than those who don't exercise. As a result, they miss fewer days of school or work. The studies have also shown that this benefit doesn't require a person to exercise really hard in a gym or fitness center. A brisk thirty-minute walk will do the trick.

Exercise and Sleep: Necessities for a Healthy Immune System

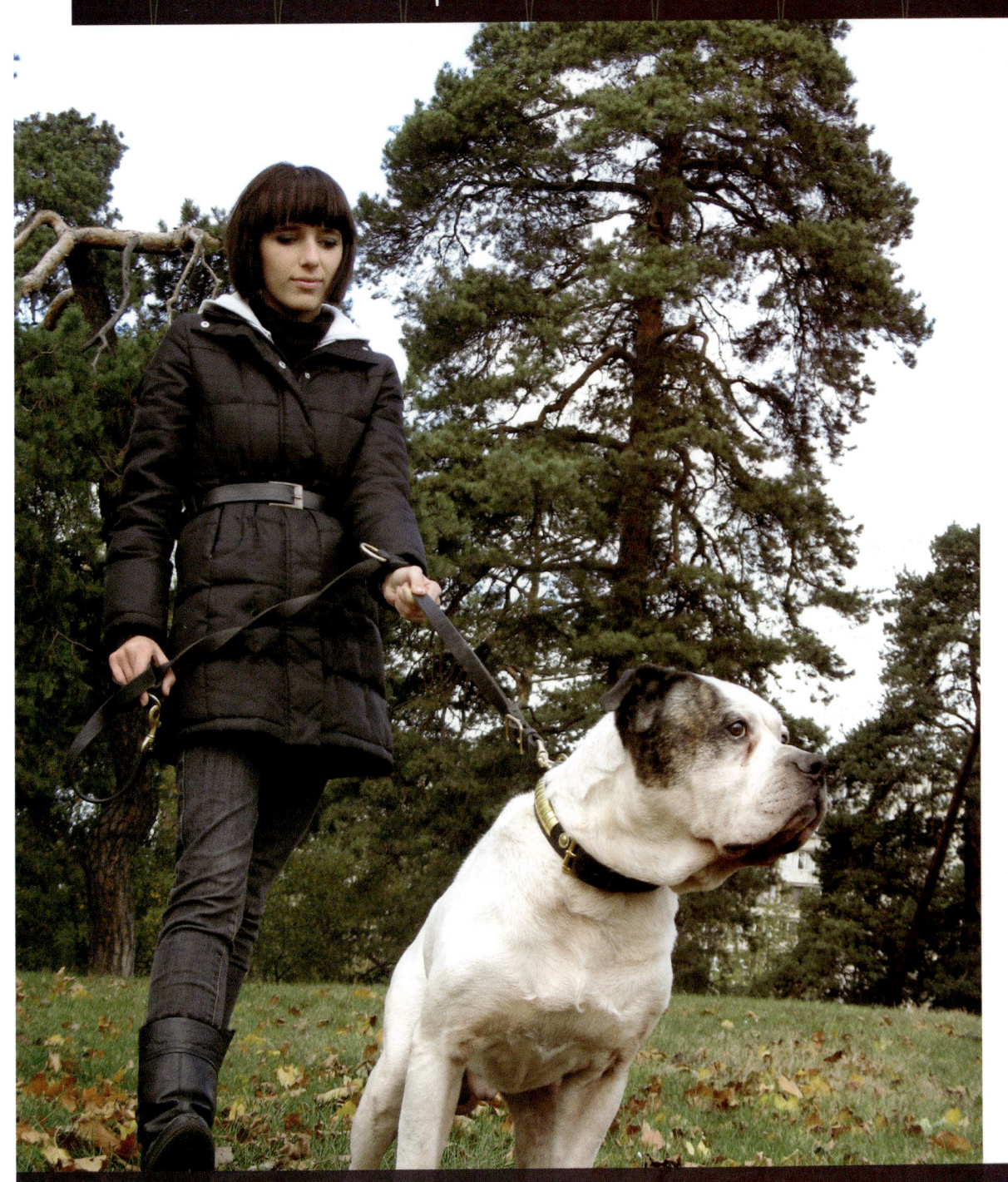

Walking a dog is great exercise for both the dog and its owner. People who exercise regularly in this manner, or any other manner, have fewer infections than do those who don't exercise.

Your Immune System: Protecting Yourself Against Infection and Illness

White blood cells, which do the work of the immune system, circulate throughout a person's body in the blood. Millions of white blood cells are also stored in the spleen, lymph nodes, and other tissues of the body. When a person exercises, his or her heart rate increases. Blood is pumped through the blood vessels faster than if the person were at rest. At the same time, white blood cells are kicked out of their storage areas and into the circulating blood. Therefore, more infection-fighting cells are available to kill invading pathogens before they can cause illness.

Exercise is also a great stress-reliever. Scientists believe this may be the most important way that exercise benefits the immune system.

Enough, but Not Too Much

If a little exercise improves the function of the immune system, does a lot of exercise help even more? The answer is no. Too much exercise can actually be harmful to the immune system. More than ninety minutes of extreme exercise can make athletes more susceptible to illness for up to seventy-two hours after the exercise. Circulating white blood cells, which increase in number in those who exercise moderately, decrease in number during extreme exercise. It takes as long as seventy-two hours for white blood cell numbers to return to normal. During this period, viruses and bacteria can invade the body and cause infections. People who run marathons, for example, exercise vigorously for more than two hours in every race. They have been shown to be six times more likely to get infections after running marathons than those who run shorter distance races.

Exercise and Sleep: Necessities for a Healthy Immune System

In a paper reported in *Exercise and Sport Sciences Reviews*, Monika Fleshner, from the Department of Integrative Physiology and the Center for Neuroscience at the University of Colorado at Boulder, sites several studies that suggest that people who exercise handle stress better and are healthier. In one study that she mentions, 364 teenage girls, all of whom were under high levels of stress, were questioned about their health. Those that rarely exercised reported more acute viral infections than those who participated in moderate exercise programs. The conclusion of the study was that physical activity may improve health by decreasing stress and its harmful effects on the immune system. Using research animals, Fleshner was able to show the ways in which exercise helps reduce stress and support immune system health.

Sleep and the Immune System

Research into the importance of sleep on health began in the 1950s. This research attracted so many scientists that a new medical subspecialty, called sleep medicine, was established in 2005. Specialists in sleep medicine are now trying to determine how sleep, or the lack of it, affects the immune system.

Some scientists believe that the immune system needs periods of sleep in order to repair itself. It takes a lot of energy in the form of calories to keep the immune system working. During the day, many of the body's organ systems compete with the immune system for energy. A teen's muscles, for instance, consume a lot of calories when he or she plays soccer. During sleep, the body has far fewer energy demands. Scientists believe that the immune system uses periods of sleep to repair itself and store up energy for use during the day.

Your Immune System: Protecting Yourself Against Infection and Illness

Getting adequate amounts of sleep is important in maintaining a healthy immune system. Scientists believe that the immune system uses periods of sleep to repair itself.

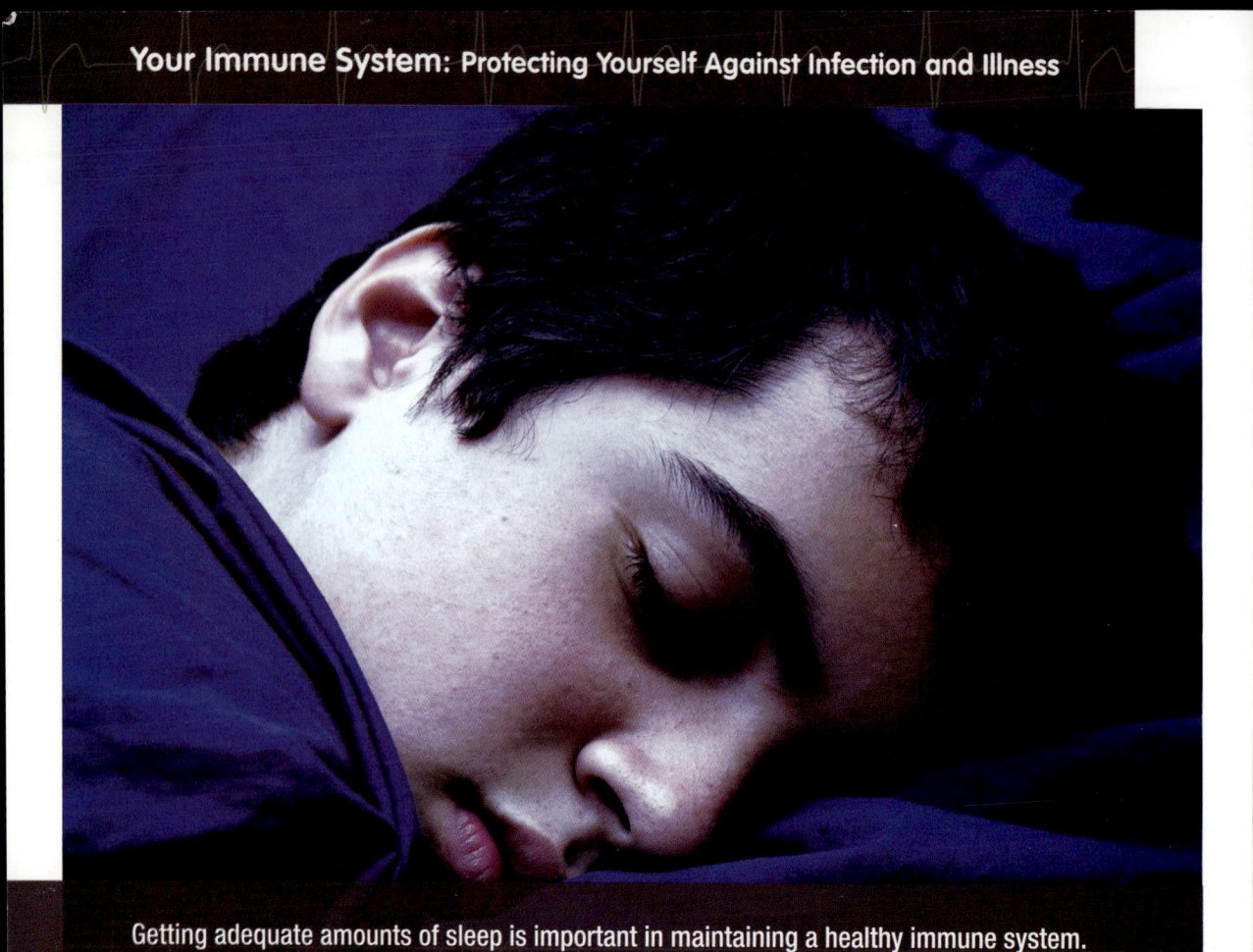

Doctors have observed that people who don't get enough sleep tend to get colds and other infections more easily than those who get normal amounts of sleep. If people who are sleep deprived are given vaccines for viruses that cause the flu, they don't make as many antibodies against the viruses as do people who get enough sleep. These and similar observations suggest that adequate sleep is essential for the normal functioning of the immune system.

The immune system also may be involved in making a person sleepy. Sleep immunologists believe that substances called "sleep factors" build up in the body throughout the day. By evening, their

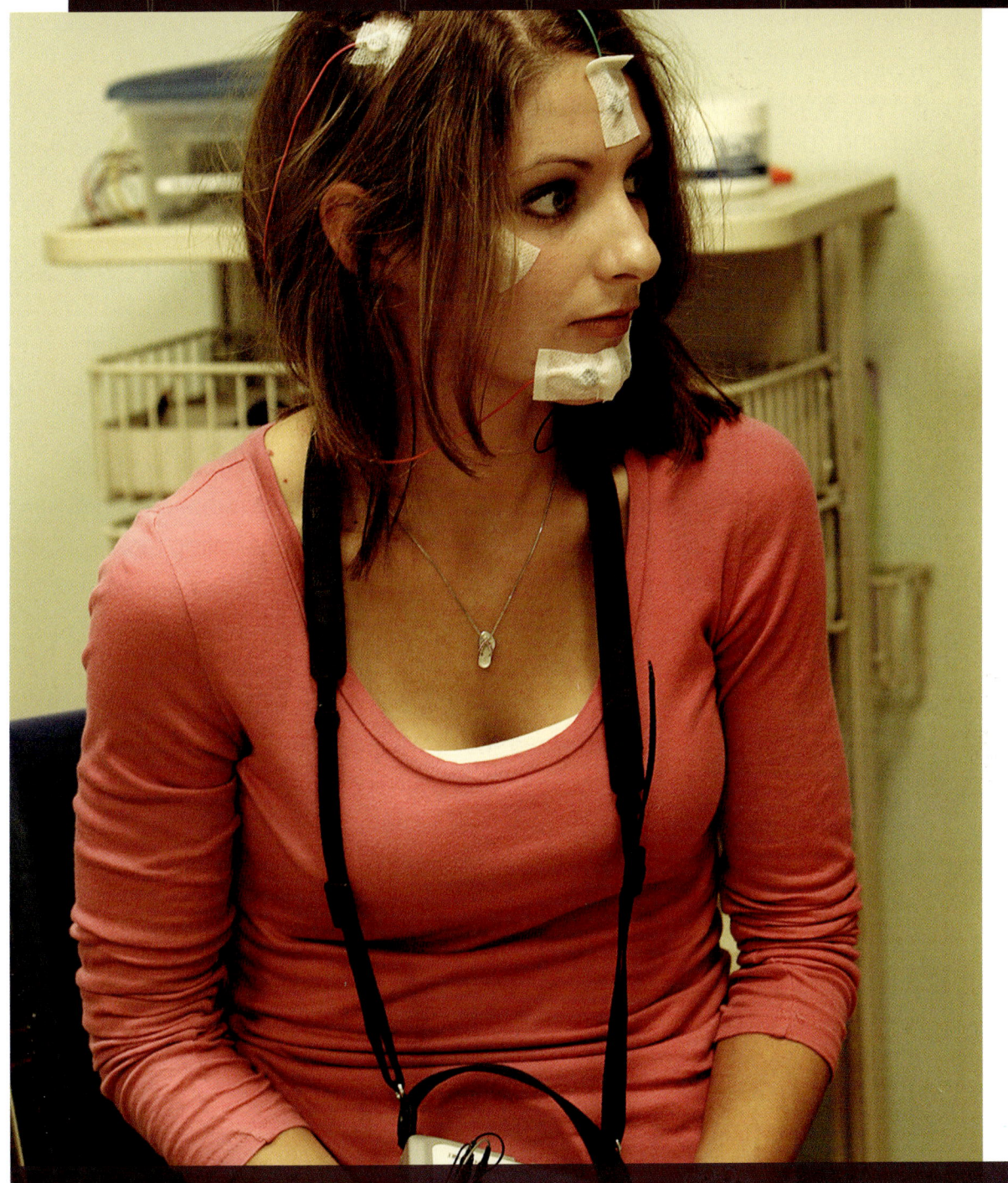

Exercise and Sleep: Necessities for a Healthy Immune System

This young woman is "wired" for a special sleep study. She has narcolepsy, a sleep disorder that may be caused by an immune system malfunction.

levels are high enough that a person feels sleepy. Cytokines are among these sleep factors. People who get infections like colds or the flu find that they are unusually sleepy. This sleepiness is probably due to the high levels of cytokines released from body cells that have been damaged by the viruses causing their illness. If sick people "listen" to their bodies and get extra sleep, they get well faster. While they sleep, their immune systems have a chance to repair and replenish themselves. As a result, they are more effective in fighting off the pathogens causing the infections.

The immune system may actually cause sleep disorders, such as narcolepsy. Narcolepsy is thought to be an autoimmune disorder. People with narcolepsy have episodes of suddenly falling asleep. They are frequently unable to drive a car or work with dangerous equipment because they never know when they will fall asleep. By studying the role of the immune system in narcolepsy and other sleep disorders, scientists may be able to develop ways to treat them.

How much sleep should a person get? Everyone's needs are different. Some people tend to need more sleep, while others need less sleep. In general, those who get at least seven or eight hours of sleep each night are the healthiest. People who get less than five to six hours of sleep are likely to become chronically sleep-deprived. Sleep deprivation may adversely affect their immune system so that they are more susceptible to illness.

Ten Great Questions to Ask a Health Professional

1. How can I tell if my immune system is functioning properly?

2. Can anything be done to enhance immunity?

3. What is the relationship between stress and immunity?

4. Can exercise improve the immune response?

5. Do I need to take vitamin and mineral supplements to protect my immune system?

6. How many hours of sleep do I need to keep my immune system healthy?

7. How does HIV affect the immune system?

8. What role does the immune system have in allergies?

9. Will I damage my immune system if I stay awake all night studying for a test?

10. What is a balanced diet and how does it affect the immune system?

Chapter 5

Lifestyle Changes That Can Protect the Immune System

Some people participate in activities that are harmful to their immune system. For example, young people who choose to smoke cigarettes or use drugs are doing significant damage to their immune system. Having unprotected sexual intercourse or using dirty needles to inject drugs may expose a person to HIV. Many adults believe that childhood is stress-free. These adults are incorrect, though. Young people experience significant stress as their bodies change and mature. They are also stressed by changing relationships, peer pressure, and school. Stress can be very harmful to the immune system if a person has not learned how to deal with stress constructively. By avoiding destructive lifestyle choices and learning how to cope with stress in a way that is healthy, a person can protect and even enhance his or her immune system.

Stress and the Immune System

A stress reaction is a group of changes that occur in a person's body in response to what are called stressors. Stressors are usually events or experiences that excite a person or cause him or her to become anxious or frightened. A pop quiz might be a stressor. Being chased by an unfriendly dog would certainly be a stressor. When faced with

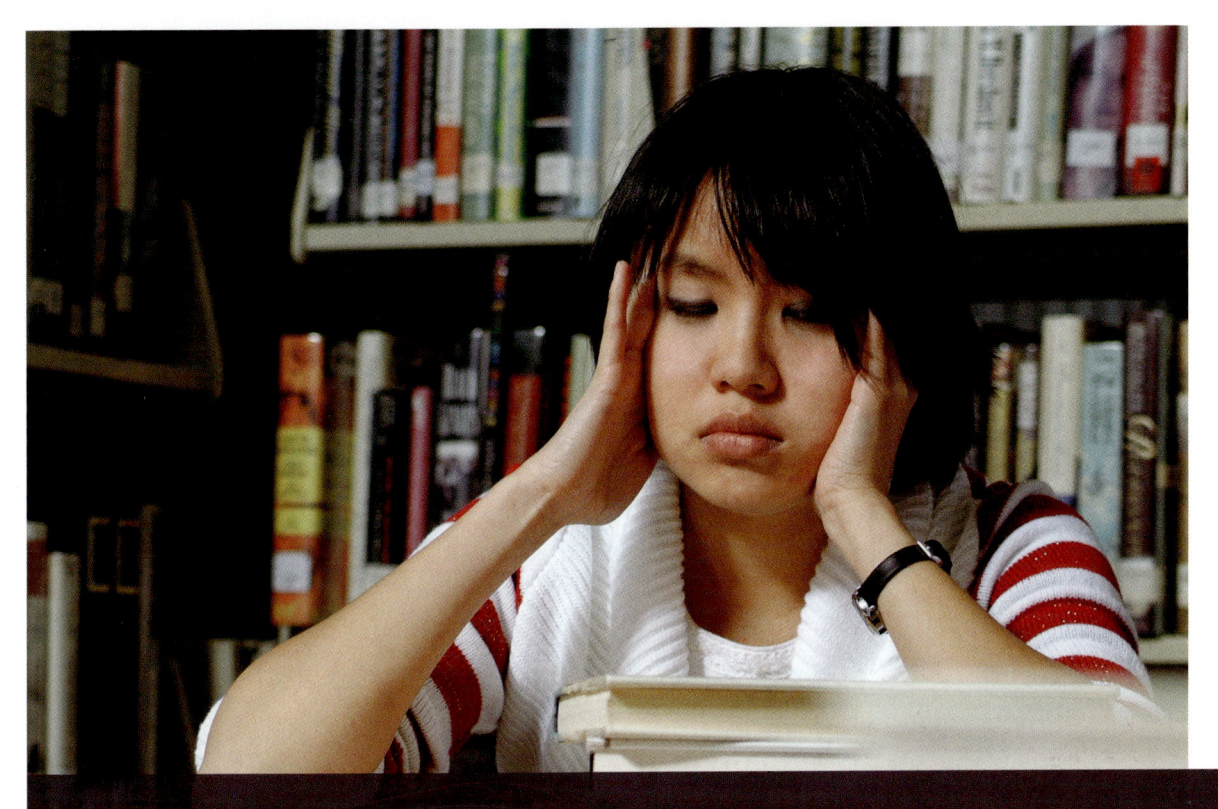

Lifestyle Changes That Can Protect the Immune System

Stress can be harmful to the immune system if a person does not deal with it constructively. Preparing lessons ahead of time is a constructive way to deal with school stressors.

stressors, people's heart rates go up, and they breathe more quickly. They may also start to sweat. These and other reactions make it possible for students to do well on tests and for mail carriers to escape from unfriendly dogs. Stress reactions involve three hormones: cortisol, epinephrine, and norepinephrine. All of these are produced in the adrenal glands, which are two small organs that sit on top of a person's kidneys. In times of stress, the hormones can turn off the inflammatory response that is produced by the innate immune system. This is a golden opportunity for pathogens that have invaded the body to start to grow and multiply.

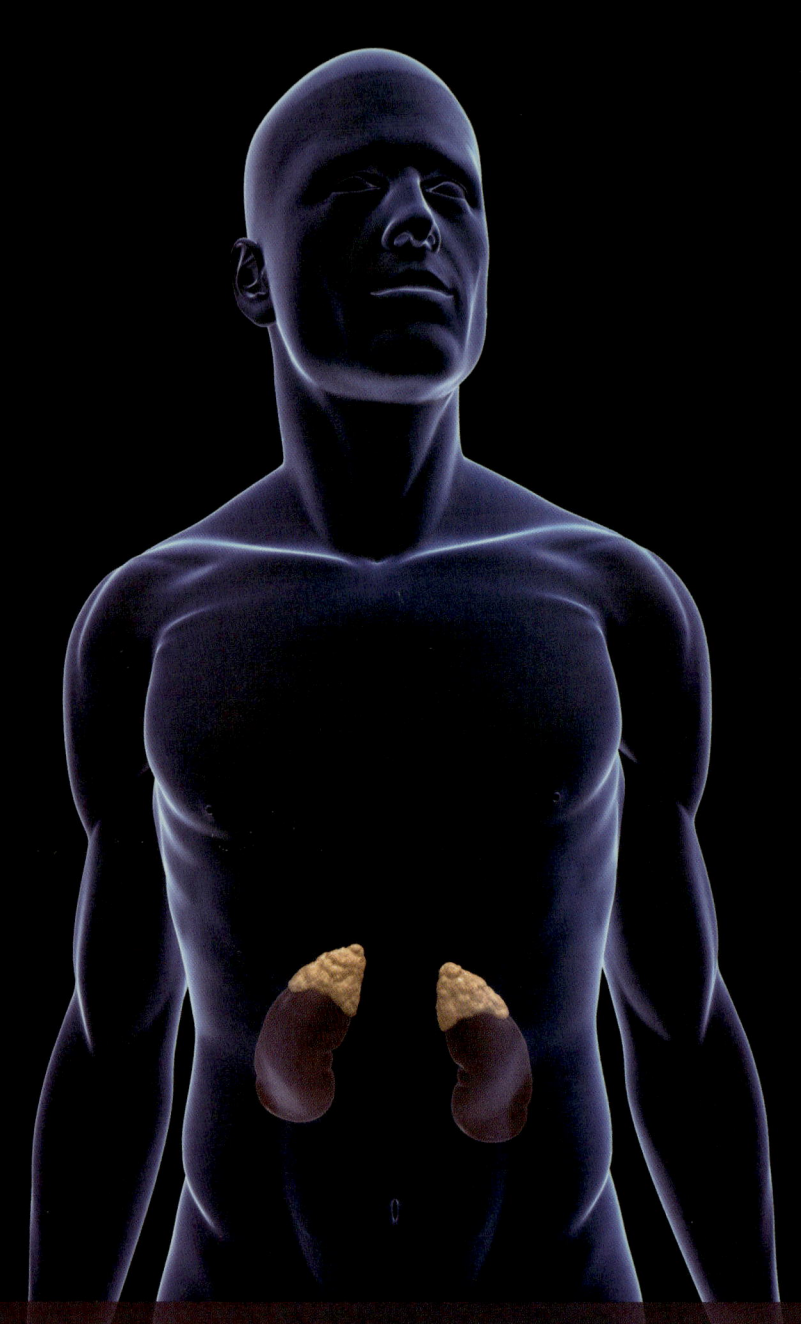

Your Immune System: Protecting Yourself Against Infection and Illness

Stress reactions involve three hormones: cortisol, epinephrine, and norepinephrine. These hormones are made in the adrenal glands, which are seen here sitting in their location atop the kidneys.

Lifestyle Changes That Can Protect the Immune System

Short-term stress does not usually create major problems for the immune system because hormone levels are only elevated for a short time. When a person is chronically stressed out, however, hormone levels are elevated for days or weeks. Immune system function is closed down. People develop infections that are caused by organisms that usually don't bother them. They may also develop very serious infections from more aggressive pathogens. It may take the immune system a long time to recover once hormone levels return to normal. An example of an infection that commonly occurs when a

Constructive Ways to Deal with Stress

People will never be without stress. In fact, life would be very dull without some stressful events. The key to keeping stress from damaging the immune system is to handle it in a positive way. Try one or more of the following activities to handle stress:

- Go for a brisk walk. Exercise is one of the best and most positive ways to deal with stress.
- Develop a routine of deep-breathing exercises.
- Try guided imagery. This involves focusing on mental images of beautiful or peaceful scenes. For example, think of a full moon shining brightly on the still water of a mountain lake.
- Do a little yoga or tai chi. These activities combine mental and physical exercise and are good stress busters.
- Experiment with expressive writing. Spend fifteen minutes writing about a stressor. Then discard the writing without reading it again.

Your Immune System: Protecting Yourself Against Infection and Illness

person is stressed out is a cold sore or fever blister on his or her lip. This infection is caused by a virus that most people have in their bodies all the time. It lurks in normal nerve cells as long as a person's immune system is functioning properly. When a person is stressed out, the virus takes advantage of the person's temporary lack of immunity to cause trouble.

Destructive Habits and the Immune System

People who smoke cigarettes and use "street drugs" (illegal drugs such as crack, cocaine, heroin, and speed) do an amazing amount of damage to their immune system. Cigarette smoke contains more than

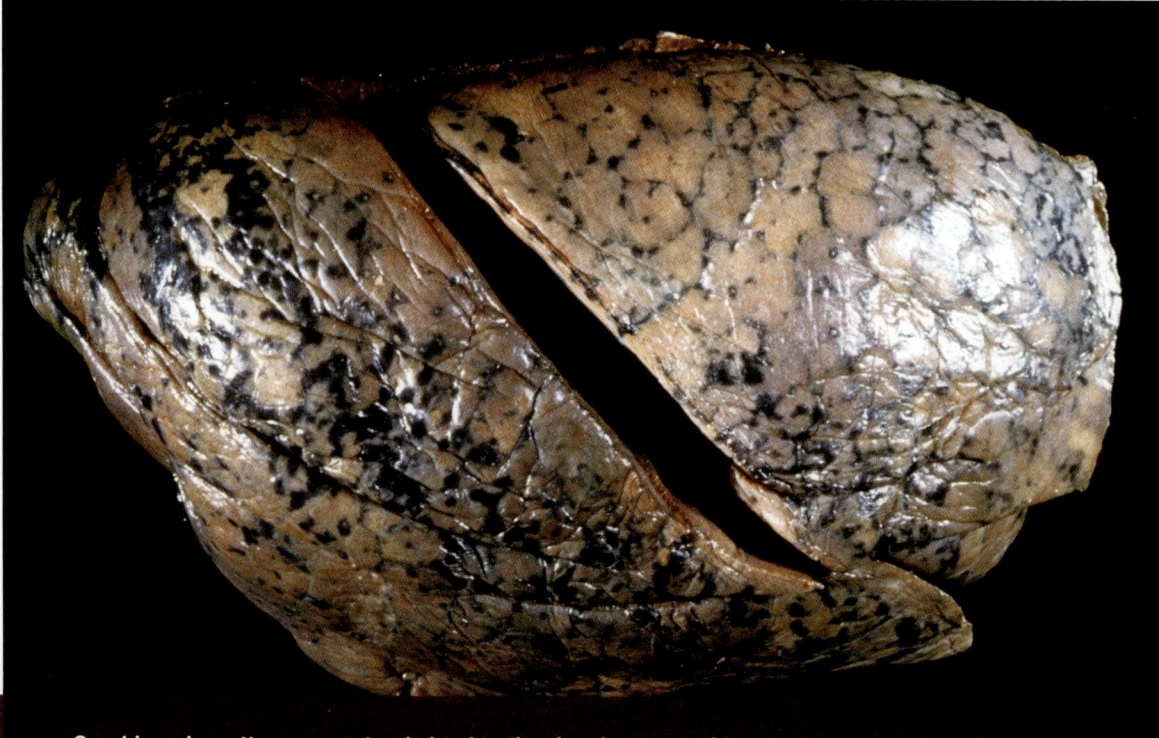

Smoking cigarettes may not only lead to the development of lung cancer, as it did in the person from whom this lung was removed, but it can also badly damage a person's immune system.

a thousand chemicals, most of which are harmful to the lungs. When smoke is inhaled, the immune cells in the nose and other parts of the respiratory system recognize that elements in smoke are foreign to the body. Innate immune responses with inflammation occur. Because smokers injure their lungs over and over again, their lungs are chronically inflamed. Their immune system is frequently overworked. White blood cells that would usually be used to fight off pathogens are instead used to consume foreign particles from smoke. This process leaves too few white blood cells in the body to prevent infections.

Street drugs have the same effect on the immune system. Impurities in the drugs cause innate immune responses with inflammation. When the drugs are injected, the risks of infection increase because the protective skin barrier is broken and pathogens are allowed to enter. Many drug abusers develop abscesses and other types of skin infections at the sites of the injections. Drug abusers may also be malnourished. This adds more stress to an already overworked and failing immune system.

HIV and AIDS

No discussion of the immune system would be complete without mentioning HIV, the virus that totally destroys the immune system. The first case of HIV and AIDS (acquired immunodeficiency syndrome) was reported in 1981. Since then, AIDS has killed more than twenty-five million people. HIV and AIDS occur in young people all over the world. AIDS is the sixth leading cause of death among fifteen- to twenty-one-year-olds in the United States. Half of all new cases of HIV infection in the United States occur in people younger than the age of twenty-five. HIV is transmitted from one person to another through the exchange of infected body fluids such as blood,

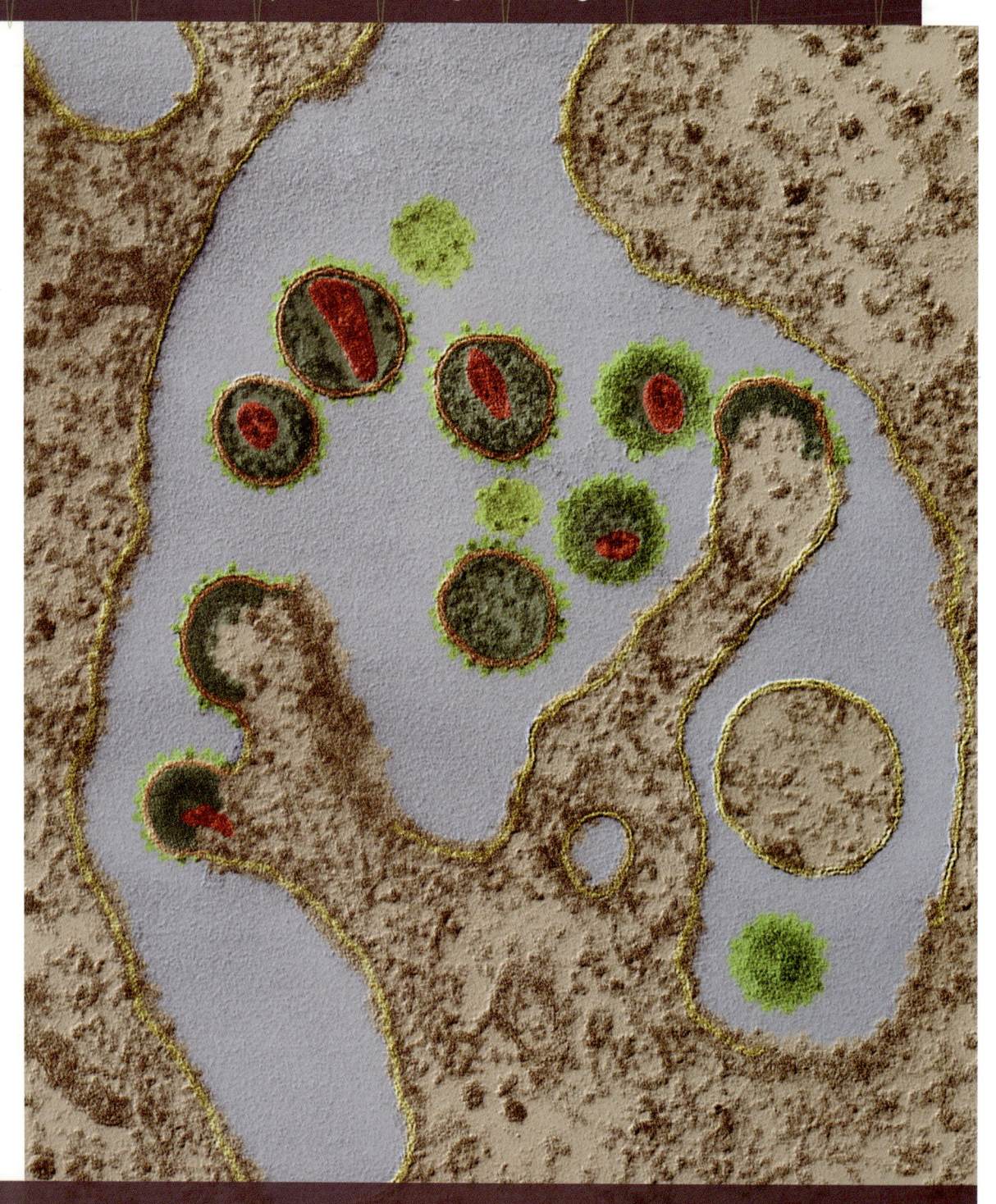

Your Immune System: Protecting Yourself Against Infection and Illness

This greatly magnified photograph of a helper T cell shows HIV particles (red and green spheres) that have invaded it. They will multiply and will eventually kill the cell.

Lifestyle Changes That Can Protect the Immune System

semen, and saliva. It can also be transmitted to unborn babies during an HIV-infected woman's pregnancy.

HIV cannot live outside the body. It depends on living cells of the host to provide the elements it needs to grow and reproduce. The cells that this particular virus invades and kills are the helper T cells of the immune system. Helper T cells are the cells that stimulate B cells and killer T cells to do their jobs. Without helper T cells to start the process, B cells don't make antibodies and killer T cells don't kill pathogens.

HIV can live hidden in an infected person's body for months or years. Although people usually experience a flulike illness shortly after they are infected, they may have no further symptoms for a long time. When HIV does come out of hiding, a person's symptoms may include fever, sore throat, cough, swollen lymph nodes in the neck, fatigue, weight loss, and purple-colored blotches on the skin. HIV infection, if untreated, eventually leads to AIDS. The diagnosis of AIDS is made when the infected person's helper T-cell count falls below one hundred and he or she develops one or more of the twenty possible associated illnesses, called AIDS-defining conditions. These conditions are frequently infections caused by unusual organisms, but they also include rare types of cancer.

In the United States, most people are well nourished and can obtain medications to suppress HIV early in their infection. Therefore, 83 percent of AIDS victims in the United States live for three years or longer. In some other countries, however, adequate nutrition and drugs to treat HIV are not as readily available. People in these countries rarely live for three years after getting HIV. Eventually, all patients with HIV develop AIDS and die of complications of the disease. Scientists are trying to develop vaccines against HIV. Because the virus mutates so rapidly, a single vaccine that will prevent all HIV infections has not been developed yet. At this time, there is no cure.

Your Immune System: Protecting Yourself Against Infection and Illness

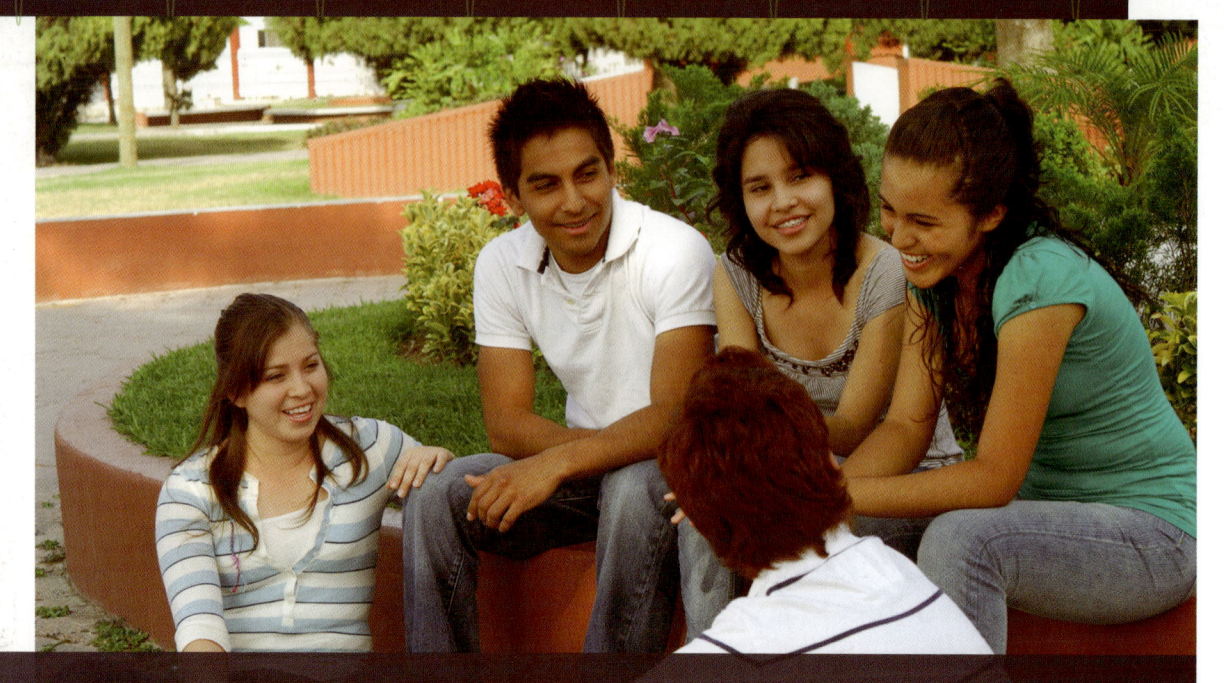

These teens can keep their immune systems healthy by eating a balanced diet, getting enough exercise and sleep, handling stressors constructively, and avoiding harmful habits and lifestyle choices.

Conclusion

The human immune system is an amazing and extremely complicated organ system. Although great strides have been made in understanding the immune system, there is still much that is not known about how it actually works. Stress and destructive habits damage the immune system. HIV and AIDS destroy it completely. The most common problems seen in people with weakened immune systems are infections. Maintaining a healthy immune system is within the power of most people who are born with a normal immune system. They just have to do what they have been told to do since childhood: Eat a balanced diet, get plenty of exercise, sleep seven to eight hours every night, handle stress constructively, and avoid harmful habits and lifestyle choices. It is a big job, but a job that is well worth the effort.

GLOSSARY

acquired immune deficiency syndrome (AIDS) A very serious, often fatal, infectious disease of the immune system that is caused by HIV.

allergen Any substance that causes an allergic reaction.

antibody A type of protein produced by the white blood cells to fight infections.

antigen A substance that is recognized by the immune system as foreign and that triggers the production of an antibody.

cancer Uncontrolled growth of cells and tissues of the body associated with progressively worsening health.

chronic Continuing for a long time or happening frequently.

diarrhea Frequent, liquid bowel movements.

disorder An illness or disease.

hormone A chemical substance produced in one place in the body and carried through the bloodstream to another part of the body, where it causes some type of reaction.

human immunodeficiency virus (HIV) The virus that causes AIDS.

impair To have a negative effect upon; to weaken or harm.

innate Inborn; existing in a person from birth.

intolerance The inability of the body to use a particular food normally. Gastrointestinal food intolerance frequently causes abdominal pain and diarrhea.

malaria A fever-producing illness that is transmitted from one person to another by bites from the anopheles mosquito. Malaria is most common in tropical countries.

malfunction The failure of something to work correctly.

malnutrition Not getting enough or the right kinds of foods to provide needed nutrients.

mutate To change or alter in appearance and/or function.

nutrient A substance that is necessary for proper metabolism in the body.

obesity A condition in which a person's weight increases beyond what is healthy because of the buildup of fat.

pathogen A disease-causing organism or virus.

philosopher A person who uses thought processes, such as reasoning and logic, to study human nature and conduct.

pollen The yellow, dustlike material shed by many plants as part of their reproductive cycle.

prescribe To order the use of.

spleen An organ, located under the ribs on the left side of the abdomen, that is a storage site for immune cells and also filters dead cells, bacteria, and other debris from the blood.

stimulate To activate, excite, or encourage.

thymus A gland that is located above and in front of the heart, where lymphocytes mature into T cells.

trigger To set off or to start.

vitamin An organic substance that occurs in foods in very small amounts. Vitamins are necessary for the normal functioning of the body.

FOR MORE INFORMATION

American Autoimmune Related Diseases Association
22100 Gratiot Avenue
East Detroit, MI 48021
(586) 776-3900
Web site: http://www.aarda.org
This organization is dedicated to the elimination of autoimmune diseases. It also works to ease suffering and the socioeconomic effects of autoimmunity through fostering education, public awareness, research, and patient services.

Canadian Society of Allergy and Clinical Immunology
774 Echo Drive
Ottawa, ON K1S 5N8
Canada
(613) 739-6272
Web site: http://www.csaci.ca
This organization is dedicated to improving the lives of people with allergies through research, support, and professional and public education.

Elton John AIDS Foundation
584 Broadway, Suite 907
New York, NY 10012
(212) 219-0670
Web site: http://www.ejaf.org
Founded by musician Sir Elton John in 1992, this organization supports innovative HIV prevention programs that try to eliminate the

stigma and discrimination associated with HIV and AIDS. It also provides direct care and support services for people living with HIV and AIDS.

Immune Deficiency Foundation
40 West Chesapeake Avenue S, Suite 308
Townsend, MD 21204
(800) 296-4433
Web site: http://www.primaryimmune.org
Since 1980, this foundation has provided accurate and timely information for people in the United States with primary immunodeficiency diseases. It provides support, education, and helps empower these individuals.

National Institute of Allergy and Infectious Disease (NIAID)
National Institutes of Health
6610 Rockledge Drive, MSC 6612
Bethesda, MD 20892-6612
(301) 496-5717
Web site: http://www3.niaid.nih.gov
The NIAID conducts and supports research on infectious, immunologic, and allergic diseases. Its Web site includes information on many diseases and excellent links to related sites.

Ontario HIV Treatment Network
1300 Yonge Street, Suite 600
Toronto, ON M4T 1X3
Canada

(416) 642-6486
Web site: http://www.ohtn.on.ca

This is a joint network of researchers, health services providers, policy makers, and community members who work together to promote excellence and innovation in HIV treatment, research, and education in the province of Ontario.

Youth AIDS
1120 Nineteenth Street NW, Suite 600
Washington, DC 20036
(202) 785-0072
Web site: http://www.psi.org

This organization, founded in 2001 by Kate Roberts, uses media, pop culture, music, theater, and sports to stop the spread of HIV and AIDS. It reaches six hundred million young people in sixty countries.

Web Sites

Due to the changing nature of Internet links, Rosen Publishing has developed an online list of Web sites related to the subject of this book. This site is updated regularly. Please use this link to access the list:

http://www.rosenlinks.com/hab/immu

FOR FURTHER READING

Anonymous. *It Happened to Nancy: By an Anonymous Teenager, A True Story from Her Diary*. Edited by Beatrice Sparks. New York, NY: HarperTeen, 2004.

Bakewell, Lisa. *Fitness Information for Teens: Health Tips About Exercise, Physical Well-Being, and Health Maintenance* (Teen Health Series). 2nd ed. Detroit, MI: Omnigraphics, Inc., 2008.

Bellenir, Karen, ed. *Allergy Information for Teens* (Teen Health Series). Detroit, MI: Omingraphics, Inc., 2006.

Bellenir, Karen. *Sleep Information for Teens* (Teen Health Series). Detroit, MI: Omnigraphics, Inc., 2007.

Bickerstaff, Linda. *Stress* (Coping in a Changing World). New York, NY: Rosen Publishing Group, 2007.

Bijlefield, Marjolijn, and Sharon Zoumbaris. *Food and You: A Guide to Health Habits for Teens*. Westport, CT: Greenwood Press, 2008.

Brice, Carleen. *Children in the Waters*. New York, NY: Ballantine, 2009.

Brown, Carrie. *The Rope Walk*. New York, NY: Pantheon, 2007.

Clark, William. *In Defense of Self: How the Immune System Really Works*. New York, NY: Oxford University Press, 2008.

Finn, Alex. *Fade to Black*. New York, NY: HarperCollins, 2006.

Fuhrman, Joel. *Disease-Proof Your Child*. New York, NY: St. Martin's Griffin, 2006.

Klosterman, Lorrie. *Immune System* (The Amazing Human Body). Tarrytown, NY: Marshall Cavendish Children's Books, 2008.

Nakazawa, Donna. *The Autoimmune Epidemic*. New York, NY: Touchstone, 2008.

For Further Reading

Robinson, Richard. *Frequently Asked Questions About AIDS and HIV* (FAQ: Teen Life). New York, NY: Rosen Publishing Group, 2008.

Rouba, Kelly. *Juvenile Arthritis: The Ultimate Teen Guide* (It Happened to Me). Lanham, MD: Scarecrow Press, 2009.

Sachs, Jessica. *Good Germs, Bad Germs: Health and Survival in a Bacterial World*. New York, NY: Hill and Wang, 2007.

Scott, Elaine. *All About Sleep from A to Zzzz*. New York, NY: Viking Juvenile, 2008.

Silvers, Cathy. *Happy Days Healthy Living: From Sitcom Teen to the Health Food Scene*. Berkeley, CA: North Atlantic Books, 2007.

Sompayrac, Lauren. *How the Immune System Works*. 3rd ed. Malden, MA: Blackwell Publishing, Inc., 2008.

BIBLIOGRAPHY

Ackerman, Tod. "Boy in Bubble Story Not Forgotten 25 Years After Death." *Houston Chronicle*, February 21, 2009. Retrieved June 3, 2009 (http://www.chron.com/disp/story.mpl/front/6274796.html).

Alagna, Magdalena. "Immune System." *Teen Health and Wellness: Real Life, Real Answers*. Rosen Publishing Group, Inc., 2009. Retrieved June 7, 2009 (http://www.teenhealthandwellness.com/article/194).

Brain, Marshall. "How Your Immune System Works." HowStuffWorks. Retrieved May 23, 2009 (http://health.howstuffworks.com/immune-system.htm).

Chandra, Ranjit Kumar. "Nutrition and the Immune System: An Introduction." *American Journal of Clinical Nutrition*, Vol. 66, No. 2, 1997, pp. 460S–463S.

Fleshner, Monika. "Physical Activity and Stress Resistance: Sympathetic Nervous System Adaptations Prevent Stress-Induced Immunosuppression." *Exercise and Sports Science Reviews*, Vol. 33, No. 3, 2005, pp.120–126.

Goodwin, Sarah. "Stress Affects Hormones Which Affect Immune System Which Alters Mental and Physical Disease." *Medical News Today*, April 19, 2004. Retrieved July 16, 2009 (http://www.medicalnewstoday.com/articles/7398.php).

Hospital Corporation of America Foundation. "Clean Hands Are Cool Hands Campaign." August 23, 2008. Retrieved September 5, 2009 (http://www.cleanhandsarecoolhand.com).

Lambert, Craig. "Deep Into Sleep." *Harvard Magazine*, July 2005. Retrieved July 16, 2009 (http://harvardmagazine.com/2005/07/deep-into-sleep.html).

Bibliography

Lim, Alvin. "Stress, Cortisol, and the Immune System: What Makes Us Get Sick?" *Science Creative Quarterly*, 2008. Retrieved July 16, 2009 (http://www.scq.ubc.ca/stress-cortisol-and-the-immune-system-what-makes-us-get-sick).

Marcos, A., E. Nova, and A. Montero. "Changes in the Immune System Are Conditioned by Nutrition." *European Journal of Clinical Nutrition*, 2003. Retrieved June 6, 2009 (http://www.nature.com/ejcn/journal/v57/n1s/full/1601819a.html).

Mayo Clinic Staff. "Primary Immunodeficiency." July 30, 2007. Retrieved May 23, 2009 (http://www.mayoclinic.com/health/primary-immunodeficiency/DS01006).

National Institute of Allergy and Infectious Diseases. "What Is a Food Allergy?" National Institutes of Health. Retrieved September 1, 2009 (http://www3.niaid.nih.gov/topics/foodAllergy).

Nemours Foundation. "Body Piercing." November 2008. Retrieved July 23, 2009 (http://kidshealth.org/teen/your_body/body_art/body_piercing_safe.html).

Nieman, David. "Does Exercise Alter Immune Function and Respiratory Infections?" *Research Digest*. President's Council on Physical Fitness and Sports, June 2001. Retrieved September 2, 2009 (http://www.fitness.gov/June2001Digest.pdf).

Quinn, Elizabeth. "Exercise and Immunity: Can Too Much Exercise Make You Sick?" January 9, 2008. Retrieved June 6, 2009 (http://sportsmedicine.about.com/od/injuryprevention/a/Ex_Immunity.htm).

Robinson, Richard. "AIDS and HIV." *Teen Health and Wellness: Real Life, Real Answers*. Rosen Publishing Group, Inc., 2009. Retrieved June 7, 2009 (http://www.teenhealthandwellness.com/article/34).

INDEX

A

acquired immune system, 12
acquired immunodeficiency syndrome (AIDS), 49–52
adrenal glands, 45
allergies, 16, 32–34, 43
amino acids, 26, 28
antibiotics, 21, 23–25, 35
antibodies, 12, 14, 15, 16, 21, 30, 32, 40, 51
antigens, 8, 9, 12, 14
autoimmune disorders, 15, 42

B

bacteria, antibiotic-resistant, 23–25
B cells, 12, 14, 32, 51
body piercing, 13
bone marrow, 4, 10, 12
"Bubble Boy," 4, 14

C

cancer, 6, 14, 16, 51
carbohydrates, 28–29
chickenpox, 22
cigarette smoking, 44, 48–49
colds, 18, 19, 36
cortisol, 45
cytokines, 10, 32, 42

D

deoxyribonucleic acid (DNA), 19
diarrhea, 34
drug use, 44, 48, 49

E

epinephrine, 45

F

Feuerbach, Ludwig, 26
Fleshner, Monika, 39
food allergies, 32–34

H

hand washing, 21, 24, 35
hay fever, 16
health professional, ten great questions to ask a, 43
histamine, 32
hormones, 45, 47
Hospital Corporation of America, 24
human immunodeficiency virus (HIV), 14, 43, 44, 49–52

I

immune system
  basics, 7–16
  and diet, 6, 14, 26–34, 36, 43, 49, 51, 52
  and exercise, 6, 36–39, 52
  and infections, 4, 6, 13, 17–25, 36, 51, 52
  and lifestyle habits, 6, 44–52
  myths and facts, 35
  and sleep, 6, 36, 39–42, 43, 52
  and stress, 6, 38–39, 43, 44–48, 52
immunodeficiency disorders, 4, 14
inflammation, 12, 13, 24, 45, 49
influenza (flu), 18, 36, 40, 51
innate immune system, 10, 12, 13, 45, 49

J

juvenile rheumatoid arthritis, 15

Index

L
lactose intolerance, 34
leukemias, 16
lymphomas, 16

M
macrophages, 9
malaria, 22
Mayo Clinic, 14
micronutrients, 29–30, 35
minerals, 29–30, 35, 43
mucus, 9, 13, 18, 19
mumps, 22
Musso, Mitchell, 24

N
narcolepsy, 42
norepinephrine, 45
nutritionists, 27, 28

O
obesity, 30–31
omega-3 fatty acids, 28
organ transplants, 8, 14

P
parasites, 4, 7, 17
pediatricians, 19
penicillin, 23
poliomyelitis, 22
pollen, 16
Popeye, 30

R
ribonucleic acid (RNA), 19

S
saturated fats, 28
Segar, Elzie Crisler, 30
severe combined immunodeficiency syndrome (SCID), 4
stress, constructively dealing with, 6, 44, 47
supplement pills, 26, 35, 43

T
T cells, 12, 21, 28, 51
thymus gland, 12
trace elements, 29–30
trans fats, 28

U
unsaturated fats, 28

V
vaccines, 21–22, 40, 51
Vetter, David Phillip, 4, 6
viral vs. bacterial infections, 19, 21
vitamins, 26, 29–30, 35, 43

W
white blood cells, 10, 12, 16, 29, 38, 49

About the Author

Linda Bickerstaff, a retired general and peripheral vascular surgeon, has cared for several teens with immune insufficiency disorders and autoimmune disorders. In spite of devastating medical and surgical problems, these young people were among the bravest and most optimistic patients she encountered in her career. They did not let their diseases control their lives. Like David Vetter, each of them contributed enormously to the knowledge of those who cared for them.

Photo Credits

Cover © www.istockphoto.com/Chadwick Reese; pp. 5, 33 © AP Images; p. 8 pttmedical/Newscom.com; p. 9 © Science Photo Library/CMSP; p. 11 © Dr. Gopal Murti/Photo Researchers, Inc.; p. 13 © www.istockphoto.com/eva serrabassa; p. 15 © Alan Sirulnikoff/Photo Researchers, Inc.; p. 18 © www.istockphoto.com/mammamaart; p. 20 Laura R. Zambuto/CDC; p. 22 Minnesota Department of Health; p. 25 David McNew/Getty Images; pp. 27, 29, 37, 46 Shutterstock.com; p. 31 Robert E. Daemmrich/Stone/Getty Images; p. 40 © www.istockphoto.com/Juanmonino; p. 41 krtphotoslive/Newscom.com; p. 45 © www.istockphoto.com/Willie B. Thomas; p. 48 © Henry Schleichkorn/CMSP; p. 50 © Eye of Science/Photo Researchers, Inc.; p. 52 © www.istockphoto.com/Carlos Martinez.

Designer: Nicole Russo; Editor: Kathy Kuhtz Campbell;
Photo Researcher: Amy Feinberg